Evidence-based
Medicine Toolkit

SECOND EDITION

D0800316

Evidence-based Medicine Toolkit

SECOND EDITION

Carl Heneghan
Centre for Evidence-based Medicine
Department of Primary Health Care
University of Oxford
Old Road Campus
Headington
Oxford
OX3 7LF

AND

Douglas Badenoch
Minervation Ltd
7200 The Quorum
Oxford Business Park North
Oxford
OX4 2JZ

Blackwell
Publishing

Blackwell Publishing Inc., 350 Main Street, Malden, Massachusetts
    02148-5020, USA
Blackwell Publishing Ltd, 9600 Garsington Road, Oxford OX4 2DQ, UK
Blackwell Publishing Asia Pty Ltd, 550 Swanston Street, Carlton, Victoria
    3053, Australia

First published 2002
Second edition 2006

5   2008

A catalogue record for this title is available from the British Library and the
Library of Congress

ISBN 978-0-7279-1841-3

Set in 8.25/10 pt Frutiger by Sparks, Oxford – www.sparks.co.uk
Printed and bound in Malaysia by Vivar Printing Sdn Bhd.

For further information on Blackwell Publishing, visit our website:
http://www.blackwellpublishing.com

Contents

*This handbook was compiled by Carl Heneghan and Douglas Badenoch.
The materials have largely been adapted from previous work by those who
know better than us, especially other members of the Centre for Evidence-
based Medicine (Chris Ball, Martin Dawes, Karin Dearness, Paul Glasziou ,
Jonathan Mant, Bob Philips, David Sackett, Sharon Straus).*

Introduction

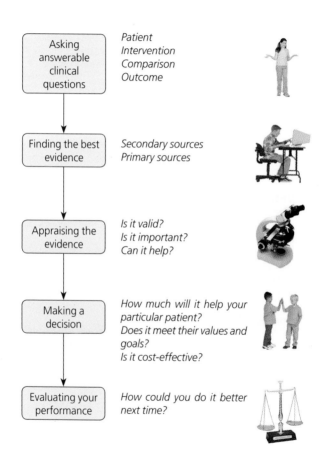

Asking answerable clinical questions
Patient
Intervention
Comparison
Outcome

Finding the best evidence
Secondary sources
Primary sources

Appraising the evidence
Is it valid?
Is it important?
Can it help?

Making a decision
How much will it help your particular patient?
Does it meet their values and goals?
Is it cost-effective?

Evaluating your performance
How could you do it better next time?

This 'toolkit' is designed as a summary and reminder of the key elements of practising evidence-based medicine (EBM). It has largely been adapted from resources developed at the Centre for Evidence-based Medicine. For more detailed coverage, you should refer to the other EBM texts and web pages cited throughout.

The first page of each chapter presents a 'minimalist' checklist of the key points. Further sections within each chapter address these points in more detail and give additional background information. Ideally, you should just need to refer to the first page to get the basics, and delve into the further sections as required.

Occasionally, you will see the dustbin icon on the right. This means that the question being discussed is a 'filter' question for critical appraisal: if the answer is not satisfactory, you should consider ditching the paper and looking elsewhere. If you don't ditch the paper, you should be aware that the effect it describes may not appear in your patient in the same way.

Definition of evidence-based medicine

Evidence-based medicine is the 'conscientious, explicit and judicious use of current best evidence in making decisions about individual patients'.

This means 'integrating individual clinical expertise with the best available external clinical evidence from systematic research' (Sackett *et al.* 2000).

We can summarize the EBM approach as a five-step model:
1 Asking answerable clinical questions.
2 Searching for the evidence.
3 Critically appraising the evidence for its validity and relevance.
4 Making a decision, by integrating the evidence with your clinical expertise and the patient's values.
5 Evaluating your performance.

Asking answerable questions

The four elements of a well-formed clinical question are:
1 **P**atient or Problem
2 **I**ntervention
3 **C**omparison intervention (if appropriate)
4 **O**utcome(s)
The terms you identify from this process will form the basis of your search for evidence and the question as your guide in assessing its relevance.

Bear in mind that how specific you are will affect the outcome of your search: general terms (such as 'heart failure') will give you a broad search, while more specific terms (for example, 'congestive heart failure') will narrow the search.

Also, you should think about alternative ways or aspects of describing your question (for example, New York Heart Association Classification).

Element	Tips	Specific example
Patient or problem	Starting with your patient ask 'How would I describe a group of patients similar to mine?'	'In women over 40 with heart failure from dilated cardiomyopathy ...'
Intervention	Ask 'Which main intervention am I considering?'	'... would adding anticoagulation with warfarin to standard heart failure therapy...'
Comparison intervention	Ask 'What is the main alternative to compare with the intervention?'	'... when compared with standard therapy alone ...'
Outcome	Ask 'What can I hope to accomplish?' or 'What could this exposure really affect?'	'... lead to lower mortality or morbidity from thromboembolism.'

Patient or problem

First, think about the patient and/or setting you are dealing with. Try to identify all of their clinical characteristics that influence the problem, which are relevant to your practice and which would affect the relevance of research you might find. It will help your search if you can be as specific as possible at this stage, but you should bear in mind that if you are too narrow in searching you may miss important articles (see next section).

Intervention

Next, think about what you are considering doing. In therapy, this may be a drug or counselling; in diagnosis it could be a test or screening programme. If your question is about harm or aetiology, it may be exposure to an environmental agent. Again, it pays to be specific when describing the intervention, as you will want to reflect what is possible in your practice. If considering drug treatment, for example, dosage and delivery should be included. Again, you can always broaden your search later if your question is too narrow.

Comparison intervention

What would you do if you didn't perform the intervention? This might be nothing, or standard care, but you should think at this stage about the alternatives. There may be useful evidence which directly compares the two interventions. Even if there isn't, this will remind you that any evidence on the intervention should be interpreted in the context of what your normal practice would be.

Outcome

There is an important distinction to be made between the outcome that is relevant to your patient or problem and the outcome measures deployed in studies. You should spend some time working out exactly what outcome is important to you, your patient, and the time-frame that is appropriate. In serious diseases it is often easy to concentrate on the mortality and miss the important aspects of morbidity. However, outcome measures, and the relevant time to their measurement, may be guided by the studies themselves and not by your original question. This is particularly true, for example, when looking at pain relief, where the patient's objective may be 'relief of pain' while the studies may define and assess this using a range of different measures.

Type of question

Once you have created a question, it is helpful to think about what type of question you are asking, as this will affect where you look for the answer and what type of research you can expect to provide the answer.

Typology for question building

Type of question	Type of evidence
Aetiology: the causes of disease and their modes of operation.	Case–control or cohort study
Diagnosis: signs, symptoms or tests for diagnosing a disorder.	Diagnostic validation study
Prognosis: the probable course of disease over time.	Inception cohort study
Therapy: selection of effective treatments which meet your patient's values.	Randomized controlled trial
Cost-effectiveness: is one intervention more cost-effective than another?	Economic evaluation
Quality of life: what will be the quality of life of the patient?	Qualitative study

Template for asking answerable clinical questions

Patient or problem	Intervention	Comparison	Outcome
List concepts here:	List concepts here:	List concepts here:	List concepts here:
Your completed clinical question:			

Deciding which question to ask:
- Which question is most important to the patient's wellbeing? (Have you taken into account the patient's perspective?)
- Which question is most feasible to answer in the time you have available?
- Which question is most likely to benefit your clinical practice?
- Which question is most interesting to you?

Further reading

Educational Prescriptions: http://www.cebm.net

Gray J. Doing the right things right. In: *Evidence Based Health-Care*. New York: Churchill Livingstone, 1997, chapter 2.

Richardson W, Wilson M, Nishikawa J, Hayward RS. The well-built clinical question: a key to evidence-based decisions [editorial]. *ACP J Club* 1995;**123**:A12–13.

Sackett DL, Rosenberg WMC, Gray JAM, Haynes RB, Richardson WS. Evidence based medicine: what it is and what it isn't. *Br Med J* 1996;**312**:71–2.

Sackett DL, Straus SE, Richardson WS, Rosenberg WMC, Haynes RB. *Evidence-Based Medicine: How to practice and teach EBM*, 2nd Edn. New York: Churchill Livingstone, 2000.

Finding the evidence: how to get the most from your searching

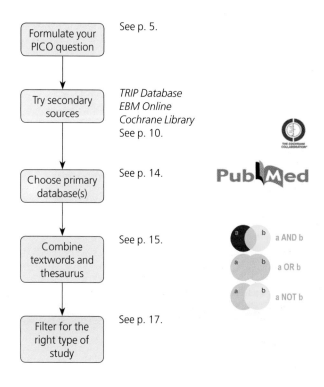

Formulate your PICO question — See p. 5.

Try secondary sources — *TRIP Database*
EBM Online
Cochrane Library
See p. 10.

Choose primary database(s) — See p. 14.

Combine textwords and thesaurus — See p. 15.

a AND b
a OR b
a NOT b

Filter for the right type of study — See p. 17.

Convert your question to a search strategy

Identify terms that you would want to include in your search:

Patient or problem	Intervention	Comparison	Outcome
Male, aged 55 Smoker Acute coronary syndrome	Low molecular weight heparin	Unfractionated heparin	Recurrence of angina, mortality

Generally, it helps you to construct a search for each concept separately, then combine them.

Think about what kind of evidence you need to answer your question:

1 Levels of evidence (see p. 94): what type of study would give you the best quality evidence for your question?
2 Secondary sources: is there a quality and relevance-filtered summary of evidence on your question, such as in *ACP Journal Club* or *Clinical Evidence*?
3 Systematic reviews: is there a systematic review in the *Cochrane Library*?
4 Bibliographic databases: in which database would you find relevant studies?

1 Try these first

TRIP Database http://www.tripdatabase.com	Use general subject terms (e.g. prostate cancer)
EBM Online http://ebm.bmjjournals.com/	Use advanced search; enter specific key words (e.g. prostatectomy)
Clinical Evidence http://www.clinicalevidence.com	Search or browse
Cochrane Library http://www.thecochranelibrary.com	Search (see p. 13)

These sources will give you the best return on your precious time.

2 Secondary sources

Of course, if someone has already searched for and appraised evidence around your question, it makes sense to use that information if possible.

Type	Description	Source
Critically appraised topics (CATs)	Appraisals of evidence in response to clinical questions	CATCrawler Journal clubs Your and your colleagues' own collection
Evidence-based summaries	Reviews of the evidence around a specific clinical topic	Bandolier, Clinical Evidence (www.clinicalevidence.com)
Structured abstracts	Appraisals of important clinical papers	EBM Online, ACP Journal clubs, evidence-based journals
Health technology assessments	Appraisals of the evidence for a specific intervention	Cochrane Library UK NHS HTA Programme
Systematic reviews	Review of all the evidence around a specific topic	Cochrane Library

A note about guidelines

An authoritative, evidence-based guideline would give you the best starting point for your search. However, we have assumed that your questions tend to be the ones that aren't answered by the guidelines. Also, it's important to bear in mind that not all guidelines are 'evidence-based' (Grimshaw 1993; Cluzeau 1999).

Good sources include:

TRIP Database	http://www.tripdatabase.com
UK National Library for Health	http://www.library.nhs.uk/
UK National Institute for Clinical Excellence	http://www.nice.org.uk/
Scottish Intercollegiate Guidelines Network	http://www.sign.ac.uk/
Canadian Medical Association	http://mdm.ca/cpgsnew/cpgs/index.asp
New Zealand Guidelines Group	http://www.nzgg.org.nz/
US National Guideline Clearinghouse	http://www.guideline.gov/

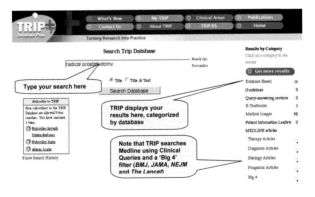

Can I trust this secondary source?

Only if you can answer 'yes' to all of the following:

- There are no conflicts of interest.
- It clearly states what question it addresses.
- There is an explicit and evidence-based methodology behind finding, producing and checking the information.
- The source is reviewed and updated regularly.

Critically appraised topics (CATs)
CATs are appraisals of the evidence found in response to a clinical question. They are a very useful way of organizing your own appraisals and sharing them with your colleagues. Many people use them to help run evidence-based journal clubs. Many people now make their CATs available on the web and you might like to start searching here. You should be wary, however, of the provenance of these CATs.

- CATmaker: http://www.cebm.net
- CAT Crawler: http://www.bii.a-star.edu.sg/research/mig/cat_search.asp

Evidence-based summaries
Evidence-based summaries are reviews of the evidence around a specific clinical topic. The findings of studies and systematic reviews are presented as answers to the clinical questions associated with that topic. However, they tend to be evidence driven (telling you what there's good evidence for) rather than question driven (telling you what you need to know).

- Clinical Evidence: http://www.clinicalevidence.com
- Bandolier: http://www.jr2.ox.ac.uk/

Structured abstracts
Secondary journals, such as *Evidence-Based Medicine*, publish structured abstracts which summarize the best quality and most clinically useful recent research from the literature. This is an excellent way to use the limited time at your disposal for reading. Recently, the BMJ have launched an 'alert' service which sends you an email when new abstracts are published that interest you.

- BMJ Updates: http://bmjupdates.mcmaster.ca/index.asp
- EBM Online: http://ebm.bmjjournals.com/

Health technology assessments (HTAs)
HTAs are assessments of the effectiveness and cost-effectiveness of health care interventions. This includes procedures, settings and programmes as well as specific drugs and equipment. The NHS HTA Programme database is included in the Cochrane Library but can be searched directly at http://www.ncchta.org/index.htm.

Systematic reviews

We'll look at SRs in more detail on p. 27. The Cochrane Library contains the full text of over 4,000 systematic reviews so it's a great place to start searching.

Note, however, that systematic reviews are found elsewhere – a recent comprehensive search for systematic reviews in cancer alone found 16,000 references (Healy 2005) – and you should search primary databases if you want to find all of the reviews in your area.

The Cochrane Library is composed of a number of different databases:

The Cochrane Database of Systematic Reviews	Full text systematic reviews prepared by the Cochrane collaboration
Database of Abstracts of Reviews of Effects (DARE)	Critical appraisal of systematic reviews published elsewhere
The Cochrane Central Register of Controlled Trials	The largest register of controlled trials in the world
The Cochrane Database of Methodology Reviews	Full-text systematic reviews of methodological studies
The Cochrane Methodology Register	A bibliography of methods used in the conduct of controlled trials
Health Technology Assessment Database	Reports of health-care interventions effectiveness
NHS Economic Evaluation Database	Economic evaluations of health-care interventions
About the Cochrane Collaboration	Methodology and background papers for the Cochrane Collaboration

Once you've done your search you can browse the results in each of these databases.

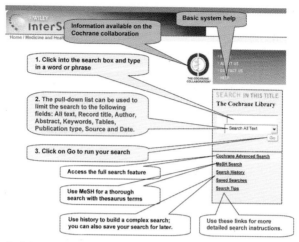

1. Click into the search box and type in a word or phrase

Information available on the Cochrane collaboration

Basic system help

2. The pull-down list can be used to limit the search to the following fields: All text, Record title, Author, Abstract, Keywords, Tables, Publication type, Source and Date.

3. Click on Go to run your search

Access the full search feature

Use MeSH for a thorough search with thesaurus terms

Use history to build a complex search; you can also save your search for later.

Use these links for more detailed search instructions.

SEARCH IN THIS TITLE
The Cochrane Library

Search All Text
Go

Cochrane Advanced Search
MeSH Search
Search History
Saved Searches
Search Tips

Use Boolean operators to combine search terms:
Use AND, OR, and NOT to create a more complex search.
Remember British and American spelling e.g. haemorrhage or hemorrhage
Use truncation*

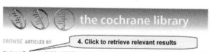

BROWSE ARTICLES BY   4. Click to retrieve relevant results

Cochrane Reviews | DARE | CENTRAL | Methodology Reviews | Methodology Register | HTA | NHS EED | About | Topics

3 Primary sources

At some point you will find yourself searching the massive collections of bibliographic records available in online databases.

Choosing the right bibliographic database(s)

Database	Coverage
CINAHL	Nursing and allied health, health education, occupational and physiotherapy, social services
MEDLINE	US database covering all aspects of clinical medicine, biological sciences, education and technology
EMBASE	European equivalent of MEDLINE, with emphasis on drugs and pharmacology
PsycLIT	Psychology, psychiatry and related disciplines, including sociology, linguistics and education

Search strategies for MEDLINE and other bibliographic databases

There are two main types of strategy for searching bibliographic databases: *thesaurus searching* and *textword searching*. You need to combine both of these to search these databases effectively.

Why do we need both of these?

Unfortunately, the index may not correspond **exactly** to your needs (and the indexers may not have been consistent in the way they assigned articles to subject headings); similarly, using textword searching alone may miss important articles. For these reasons, you should use **both** thesaurus and textword searching.

Most databases allow you to build up a query by typing multiple statements, which you can combine using Boolean operators (see below). Here is an example from PubMed (www.pubmed.gov).

Question: In patients who have had a heart attack, does simvastatin reduce mortality?

Patient or problem	Intervention	Comparison	Outcome
Heart attack/ myocardial infarction	Simvastatin	Standard care	Mortality

Textword search	Thesaurus search
#1 myocardial AND infarct*	#2 'Myocardial infarction'[MeSH]
#3 heart AND attack*	
#4 #1 OR #2 OR #3: *yields 136,950 documents about myocardial infarction*	
#5 simvastatin*	#6 'Simvastatin'[MeSH]
#7 #5 OR #6: *yields 3,206 documents about simvastatin*	
#8 #4 AND #7: *yields 191 documents about myocardial infarction and simvastatin*	

You will have noticed as you went along that the textword and thesaurus searches for each term yielded different sets of results. This underlines the importance of using both methods. It is best to start your search by casting your net wide with both textword and thesaurus searching and progressively narrowing it to by adding more specific terms or limits.

Specific notes on PubMed
Unfortunately, different database vendors implement these features differently. In PubMed, typing a single term into the search box automatically carries out both a textword and thesaurus search. You can check how exactly it has searched using 'Details' tab.

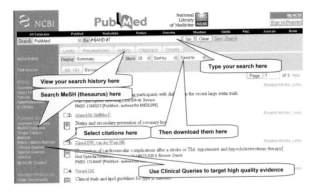

To increase **sensitivity**:
1 Expand your search using (broader terms in) the *thesaurus*.
2 Use a *textword* search of the database.
3 Use *truncation* and *wildcards* to catch spelling variants.
4 Use *Boolean* OR to make sure you have included all alternatives for the terms you are after (for example (myocardial AND infarction) OR (heart AND attack)).

To increase **specificity**:
1 Use a *thesaurus* to identify more specific headings.
2 Use more specific terms in *textword* search.
3 Use *Boolean* AND to represent other aspects of the question.
4 *Limit* the search by publication type, year of publication, etc.

Depending on which databases you use, these features might have different keystrokes or commands associated with them; however, we have tried to summarize them as best we can in the table below.

Feature key explanation

Expand thesaurus	Use *explosion* and *include all sub-headings* to (MeSH) expand your search.
Truncation *(or $)*	analy*, analysis, analytic, analytical, analyse, etc.
Wildcards?	gyn?ecology, gynaecology, gynecology; randomi?*, randomization, randomization, randomized.
Boolean AND	Article must include both terms.
OR	Article can include either term.
NOT	Excludes articles containing the term (for example econom* NOT economy picks up economic and economical but not economy).
Proximity NEAR	Terms must occur close to each other (for example within 6 words) (heart NEAR failure).
Limit (variable)	As appropriate, restrict by publication type (clinicaltrial. pt), year, language, possibly by study characteristics, or by searching for terms in specific parts of the document (for example diabet* in ti will search for articles which have diabetes or diabetic in the title).
Related articles	Once you've found a useful article, this feature (for example in PubMed by clicking the 'Related' hyperlink) searches for similar items in the database.

4 Targeting high-quality evidence

If you want to target high-quality evidence, it is possible to use search strategies that will only pick up the best evidence; see the SIGN webiste for examples for the main bibliographic databases (http://www.sign.ac.uk/methodoglogy/filters.html).

Some MEDLINE services provide such search 'filters' online, so that you can click them or upload them automatically. The PubMed Clinical Queries feature allows you to target good quality diagnosis, prognosis, aetiology and therapy articles as well as systematic reviews.

Searching the internet
You might like to begin searching the internet using a specialized search engine which focuses on evidence-based sources. Two such services are TRIP (see above) and SUMSearch (http://sumsearch. uthscsa.edu/searchform45.htm) which search other websites for you, optimizing your search by question type and number of hits.

AskMedline is a new service which allows you to search Medline using the PICO structure: http://askmedline.nlm.nih.gov/ask/pico. php

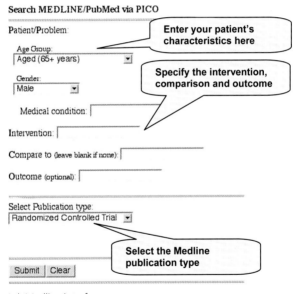

Ask Medline interface

Search engines

Generic internet search engines such as Google are very effective search tools, providing you with a relevance-ranked list of hits.

Some hints to help you get the most out of search engines:

- Use multiple terms to increase the specificity of your search;
- Google automatically truncates search terms and ignores common words such as 'where' and 'how'
- Use quotes to indicate phrases (e.g. 'myocardial infarction');
- Use the minus sign to show terms you don't want to find (e.g. hospital –drama if you want to find hospitals but not hospital dramas)
- Use the advanced search if you want better results;
- Be prepared to look at more than the first page of results.

However, you should be wary of relying on internet search engines because:

- relevance ranking is based on characteristics of the web page, not on an assessment of what it's about (as is the case with MeSH);
- it is not comprehensive;
- you cannot compile complex searches as in bibliographic databases;
- many large web sites contain 'deep content' which is not indexed by search engines.

Can this web site help you to answer your question?

There are many large web sites which provide detailed information about health care topics; sometimes you may be asked to recommend a site for a patient to read up on their condition. But how can you tell when a site is any good?

1 Is the site accessible to disabled users?

2 Is the design clear and transparent?

3 Can you use it effectively?

4 Are the objectives of the site and its provider clearly stated?

5 Are there any conflicts of interest?

6 Is it up to date?

7 Does the site report a content production method which includes systematic searching, appraisal and evaluation of information (Badenoch 2004)?

Further reading

Ask Medline: http://askmedline.nlm.nih.gov/ask/pico.php

CASP. Evidence-Based Health Care (CD-ROM and Workbook). Oxford: Update Software, 2005.

SIGN Search Filters: http://www.sign.ac.uk/methodology/filters.html

McKibbon A. *PDQ Evidence-Based Principles and Practice*. Hamilton, ON: BC Decker, 2000.

PubMed: http://www.pubmed.gov

The SCHARR guide to EBP on the internet: http://www.shef.ac.uk/scharr/ir/netting/.

SUMSearch: http://sumsearch.uthscsa.edu/

TRIPDatabase: http://www.tripdatabase.com

Badenoch DS, Holland J, Hunt D, Massart R, Tomlin A. The LIDA Tool: Minervation validation instrument for health care web sites. Oxford: Minervation Ltd, 2004.

Grimshaw J, Russell I. Effect of clinical guidelines on medical practice: a systemic review of rigorous evaluations. *Lancet* 1993;**242**:1317–22.

Cluzeau FA, Littlejohns P, Grimshaw JM, Feder G, Moran SE. Development and application of a generic methodology to assess the quality of clinical guidelines. *Int J Qual Health Care* 1999;**11**:21–8.

Healy G. Systematic reviews in cancer: results of a comprehensive search. Oxford: Minervation/NLH Cancer Specialist Library, 2005.

Critical appraisal of guidelines

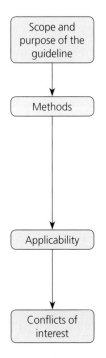

Scope and purpose of the guideline

1 Does the guideline address a clear issue?
2 Are the target users of the guideline clearly defined?

Methods

3 Was there a comprehensive search for the evidence?
4 Are the criteria for data extraction clearly described?
5 Are the methods used for formulating the recommendations clearly described?
6 Are the health benefits, side effects and risks of the interventions considered in formulating recommendations?

Applicability

7 Are different options for diagnosis and/or treatment of the condition clearly presented?
8 Are the key recommendations identifiable?

Conflicts of interest

9 Is the guideline editorially independent from the funding body?
10 Are the conflicts of interest of the developing members recorded?
11 How up to date is the guideline?

Scope and purpose of the guideline

The main benefit of guidelines is to improve the quality of care received by patients. They are an increasingly familiar part of clinical practice and have the potential not only to benefit patients but also to harm.

Possible reasons for this are:

- Evidence about what to recommend is often missing, misleading, or misinterpreted.
- Developers may lack the skills ands resources to examine all the evidence.
- Recommendations can be influenced by the opinions, experience and composition of the development group.
- Interventions that experts believe are good for patients may be inferior to other options, ineffective, or even harmful.

The purpose of appraising guidelines is to weigh up the extent to which these biases may be a problem.

1 Does the guideline address a clear issue?

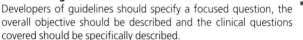

Developers of guidelines should specify a focused question, the overall objective should be described and the clinical questions covered should be specifically described.

It should be easy to tell which patients the guideline applies to; their views and preferences should have been sought in the development process.

2 Are the target users of the guideline clearly defined?

You should ensure the purpose of the guideline meets the use you intend for it.

Guidelines may be disseminated to assist health professionals with clinical decision making (e.g. clinical algorithms and reminders), to facilitate evaluation of practices (e.g. utilization review, quality assurance), or to set limits on health resource choices. Guidelines may be directed at different practitioners and different settings.

Methods

3 Was there a comprehensive search for the evidence?

The search for evidence should be as comprehensive as a systematic review (see p. 29). Multiple databases should be used and key stakeholders should be identified for further information.

4 Are the criteria for selecting and combining the evidence clearly described?

There should be a clear and explicit statement of appropriate inclusion and exclusion criteria which were applied to the evidence.

Guideline developers should consider all reasonable practice options, and all important potential outcomes. You should look for information on morbidity, mortality, and quality of life associated with each option.

In examining cost-effectiveness outcomes, consider the perspective the developers have taken (see p. 70). This may influence final recommendations. It may be difficult for you to determine whether their cost estimates are valid or applicable for your practice setting.

5 Are the methods used for formulating the recommendations clearly described?

Guideline developers often deal with inadequate evidence; therefore, they may have to consider a variety of studies as well as reports of expert and consumer experience.

There must be clarity about the type and quantity of evidence upon which each recommendation is based.

Look for a report of methods used to synthesize preferences from multiple sources. Informal and unstructured processes to judge values may be susceptible to undue influence by individual panel members, particularly the panel chair. Appropriate, structured, processes, such as the Delphi method (opposite) increase the likelihood that all important values are duly considered.

You should determine whether and how expert opinion was used to fill in gaps in the evidence.

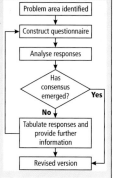

6 Are the health benefits, side effects and risks of the interventions considered in formulating recommendations?

The clinical problems for which guidelines are needed often involve complex tradeoffs between competing benefits, harms and costs, usually under conditions of ambiguity. Even with evidence from randomized clinical trials, the effect size of an intervention may be marginal or the intervention may be associated with costs, discomforts, or impracticalities that lead to disagreement or ambivalence among guideline developers about what to recommend. Recommendations may differ depending on our relative emphasis on specific benefits, harms and costs.

It is particularly important to know how patient preferences were considered. Methods for directly assessing patient and societal values exist but are rarely used by guideline developers. You should look for information that must be obtained from and provided to patients and for patient preferences that should be considered. It is important to consider whether the values assigned (implicitly or explicitly) to alternative outcomes could differ enough from your patients' preferences to change a decision about whether to adopt a recommendation.

Applicability

7 Are different options for diagnosis and/or treatment of the condition clearly presented?

To be really useful, guidelines should describe interventions well enough for their exact duplication. You must determine whether your patients are the intended target of a particular guideline. If your patients have a different prevalence of disease or risk factors, for instance, the guidelines may not apply.

8 Are the key recommendations identifiable?

To be useful, recommendations should give practical, unambiguous advice about a specific health problem. The practice guideline should convince you that the benefits of following the recommendations are worth the expected harms and costs.

The 'strength' or 'grade' of a recommendation (see p. 94) should be informed by multiple considerations:

(i) the quality of the investigations which provide the evidence for the recommendations;

(ii) the magnitude and consistency of positive outcomes relative to negative outcomes (adverse effects, burdens to the patient and the health care system, costs); and

(iii) the relative value placed upon different outcomes.

It is very important for you to scrutinize a guideline document for what, in addition to evidence, determines the wording of the recommendations.

Inferring strength of evidence from study design alone may overlook other determinants of the quality of evidence, such as sample size, recruitment bias, losses to follow-up, unmasked outcome assessment, atypical patient groups, irreproducible interventions, impractical clinical settings, and other threats to internal and external validity.

Conflict of interest
9 Is the guideline editorially independent from the funding body?

Expert panels and consensus groups are often used to determine what a guideline will say. By identifying the agencies that have sponsored and funded guideline development, you can decide whether their interests or delegates are over-represented on the consensus committee.

10 Are the conflicts of interest of the developing members recorded?

Panels dominated by members of speciality groups may be subject to intellectual, territorial, and even financial biases (some organizations screen potential panel members for conflicts of interest, others do not).

Panels which include a balance of research methodologists, practising generalists and specialists, and public representatives are more likely to have considered diverse views in their deliberations.

11 How up to date is the guideline?

You should look for two important dates:

(i) the publication date of the most recent evidence considered;

(ii) the date on which the final recommendations were made.

Some guidelines also identify studies in progress and new information that could change the guideline. Ideally, these considerations may be used to qualify guidelines as 'temporary' or 'provisional,' to specify dates for expiration or review, or to identify key research priorities. You should consider how likely it is that important evidence has been published since the guideline, which might affect your decision.

Further reading

The AGREE Collaboration: Appraisal of Guidelines for Research and Evaluation (AGREE) Instrument, 2001. http://www.agreecollaboration.org

Grimshaw J, Russell I. Effect of clinical guidelines on medical practice: a systemic review of rigorous evaluations. *Lancet* 1993;**242**:1317–22.

Cluzeau FA, Littlejohns P Grimshaw JM Feder G Moran SE. Development and application of a generic methodology to assess the quality of clinical guidelines. *Int J Qual Health Care* 1999;**11**:21–8.

Appraising systematic reviews

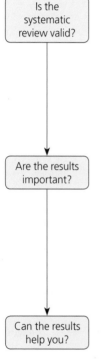

Is the systematic review valid?

Are the results important?

Can the results help you?

1 Is it a systematic review of high-quality studies which are relevant to your question?

2 Does the methods section adequately describe:
  • a comprehensive search for all the relevant studies?
  • how the reviewers assessed the validity of each study?

3 Are the studies consistent, both clinically and statistically?

Are they clinically significant?
If the review reports odds ratios (ORs), you can generate an NNT if you have an estimate of your patient's expected event rate (PEER).

$$NNT = \frac{1 - \{PEER \times (1 - OR)\}}{(1 - PEER) \times PEER \times (1 - OR)}$$

How precise are the results?

See p. 31.

Is the systematic review valid?

> **A systematic review** is 'a review of a clearly formulated question that uses systematic and explicit methods to identify, select and critically appraise relevant research, and to collect and analyse data from studies that are included in the review. Statistical methods may or may not be used to analyse and summarize the results of the included studies' (Cochrane Library, Glossary).
>
> Three key features of such a review are:
>
> - a strenuous effort to locate all original reports on the topic of interest
> - critical evaluation of the reports
> - conclusions are drawn based on a synthesis of studies which meet pre-set quality criteria
>
> When synthesizing results, a meta-analysis may be undertaken. This is 'the use of statistical techniques in a systematic review to integrate the results of the included studies' (Cochrane Library, Glossary), which means that the authors have attempted to synthesize the different results into one overall statistic.
>
> The best source of systematic reviews is the Cochrane Library, available by subscription on CD or via the internet. Many of the systematic reviews so far completed are based on evidence of effectiveness of an intervention from randomized controlled trials (RCTs).

1 Is it a systematic review of the right type of studies which are relevant to your question?

Only if:
- The review addresses a clearly defined question which is relevant to you,
- The review includes studies which also look at this question,
- The studies are the right design to address this question (see p. 5).

Reviews of poor-quality studies simply compound the problems of poor-quality individual studies. Sometimes, reviews combine the results of variable-quality trials (for example randomized and quasi-randomized trials in therapy); the authors should provide separate information on the subset of randomized trials.

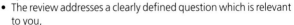

2 Does the methods section describe how all the relevant trials were found and assessed?

The paper should give a comprehensive account of the sources consulted in the search for relevant papers, the search strategy used to find them, **and** the quality and relevance criteria used to decide whether to include them in the review.

Search strategy
Some questions you can ask about the search strategy:
- The authors should include hand searching of journals and searching for unpublished literature.
- Were any obvious databases missed?
- Did the authors check the reference lists of articles and of text-books (citation indexing)?
- Did they contact experts (to get their list of references checked for completeness and to try and find out about ongoing or un-published research)?
- Did they use an appropriate search strategy: were important subject terms missed?

Did the authors assess the trials' validity?
You should look for a statement of how the trials' validity was assessed. Ideally, two or more investigators should have applied these criteria independently and achieved good agreement in their results.

Publication bias

The reviewers' search should aim to minimize **publication bias:** the tendency for negative results to be unequally reported in the literature. The importance of a clear statement of inclusion criteria is that studies should be selected on the basis of these criteria (that is, any study that matches these criteria is included) rather than selecting the study on the basis of the results.

What criteria were used to extract data from the studies?
Again, it's helpful to think in terms of patient, intervention, out-come:
- Who were the study participants and how is their disease status defined?

- What intervention/s were given, how and in what setting?
- How were outcomes assessed?

A point to consider is that the narrower the inclusion criteria, the less generalizable are the results. However, if inclusion criteria are too broad heterogeneity (see below) becomes an issue.

3 Are the studies consistent, both clinically and statistically?

You have to use your clinical knowledge to decide whether the groups of patients, interventions, and outcome measures were similar enough to merit combining their results. If not, this **clinical heterogeneity** would invalidate the review.

Similarly, you would question the review's validity if the trials' results contradicted each other. Unless this **statistical hetero-geneity** can be explained satisfactorily (such as by differences in patients, dosage, or durations of treatment), this should lead you to be very cautious about believing any overall conclusion from the review.

Are the results important?

Because systematic reviews usually examine lots of different re-sults, the first step is for you to consider which patient group, in-tervention and outcome matters most to you.

The most useful way of interrogating the results of systematic reviews is to look at the figures, illustrated below.

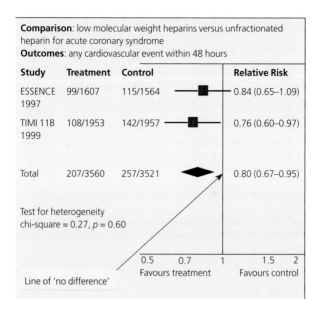

Comparison: low molecular weight heparins versus unfractionated heparin for acute coronary syndrome
Outcomes: any cardiovascular event within 48 hours

Study	Treatment	Control		Relative Risk
ESSENCE 1997	99/1607	115/1564		0.84 (0.65–1.09)
TIMI 11B 1999	108/1953	142/1957		0.76 (0.60–0.97)
Total	207/3560	257/3521		0.80 (0.67–0.95)

Test for heterogeneity
chi-square = 0.27, $p = 0.60$

0.5   0.7   1   1.5   2
Favours treatment   Favours control

Line of 'no difference'

The top of the diagram tells you which PICO question is being analysed. Use this to select the graph/s that matter to you.

This is a meta-analysis of two studies: ESSENCE 1998 and TIMI 1999. Their individual results are shown by the blue squares. Note that each of these squares has a horizontal line to show you the confidence interval for that outcome in that study.

The black diamond tells you the combined result (Relative Risk = 0.80); the width of the diamond tells you the combined confidence interval (0.67 to 0.95). Because the diamond doesn't cross the 'line of no difference', the result is statistically significant.

Odds: what they are and why they're used

In measuring the efficacy of a therapy, odds can be used to describe risk. The odds of an event are the probability of it occurring compared to the probability of it not occurring. So, odds of 1 means that an event has a 50/50 (or 50%) chance of occurring.

Statisticians like odds because they are more amenable to meta-analytic techniques than other measures of risk.

Is this odds ratio or relative risk clinically important?

Because odds ratios and relative risks are *relative* measures of efficacy, they can't tell us how many patients are likely to be helped by the regimen. We need absolute measures of benefit to derive an NNT.

To do this, we need to get an estimate of baseline risk (or odds), then multiply that by the relative risk (or odds ratio) from the review.

For more help with this, see http://www.cebm.net and p. 74 on applying the evidence to particular patients.

Logarithmic odds

Odds ratios are usually plotted on a log scale to give an equal line length on either side of the line of 'no difference'. If odds ratios are plotted on a log scale, then a log odds ratio of 0 means no effect, and whether or not the 95% confidence interval crosses a vertical line through zero will lead to a decision about its significance.

Binary or continuous data

Binary data (an event rate: something that either happens or not, such as numbers of patients improved or not) is usually combined using odds ratios. Continuous data (such as numbers of days, peak expiratory flow rate) is combined using differences in mean values for treatment and control groups (weighted mean differences or WMD) when units of measurement are the same, or standardized mean differences when units of measurement differ. Here the difference in means is divided by the pooled standard deviation.

How precise are the results?
The statistical significance of the results will depend on the extent of any confidence limits around the result (see p. 31). The review should include confidence intervals for all results, both of individual studies and any meta-analysis.

Further reading
Altman D. *Practical Statistics for Medical Research*. Edinburgh: Churchill Livingstone, 1991.

Antman EM, Lau J, Kupelnick B, Mosteller F, Chalmers TC. A comparison of results of metaanalyses of randomized control trials and recommendations of clinical experts. *J Am Med Assoc* 1992;**268**:240–8.

Cohen M, Demers C, Gurfinkel EP *et al*. Low-molecular-weight heparins in non-ST-segment elevation ischemia: the ESSENCE trial. Efficacy and safety of subcutaneous enoxaparin versus intravenous unfractionated heparin, in non-Q-wave coronary events. *Am J Cardiol* 1998;**82**(5B):19L–24L.

Glasziou P. *Systematic Reviews in Health Care: A practical guide*. Cambridge: Cambridge University Press, 2001.

NHS Centre for Reviews and Dissemination: http://www.york.ac.uk/inst/crd/

Oxman AD, Cook DJ, Guyatt GH, for the Evidence-Based Medicine Working Group. Users' Guides to the Medical Literature VI: How to use an overview. *J Am Med Assoc* 1994;**272**(17):1367–71.

Sackett DL, Straus SE, Richardson WS, Rosenberg WMC, Haynes RB. *Evidence-Based Medicine: How to practice and teach EBM*, 2nd Edn. New York: Churchill Livingstone, 2000.

Seers K. Systematic review. In: Dawes M, Davies P, Gray A, Mant J, Seers K, Snowball R (eds) *Evidence-Based Practice: A primer for health care professionals*. Edinburgh: Churchill Livingstone, 1999, pp. 85–100.

Antman EM, McCabe CH, Gurfinkel EP, Turpie AG, Bernink PJ, Salein D, Bayes De Luna A, Fox K, Lablanche JM, Radley D, Premmereur J, Braunwald E. Enoxaparin prevents death and cardiac ischemic events in unstable angina/non-Q-wave myocardial infarction. Results of the thrombolysis in myocardial infarction (TIMI) 11B trial. *Circulation* 1999;**100**(15):1593–601.

Appraising diagnosis articles

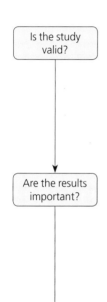

Is the study valid?

1 Was there a clearly defined question?
2 Was the presence or absence of the target disorder confirmed with a reference standard?
  • Was this comparison independent from and blind to the study test results?
3 Was the test evaluated on an appropriate spectrum of patients?
4 Was the reference standard applied to all patients?

Are the results important?

Work out sensitivity, specificity and likelihood ratios (LRs):

		Target disorder	
		Present	**Absent**
Test result	**Positive**	a	b
	Negative	c	d

$$\text{Sensitivity} = \frac{a}{a + c}$$

$$\text{Specificity} = \frac{b}{b + d}$$

$$\begin{array}{l}\text{LR+} \\ \text{(positive result)}\end{array} = \frac{\text{sensitivity}}{(1 - \text{specificity})}$$

$$\begin{array}{l}\text{LR−} \\ \text{(negative result)}\end{array} = \frac{(1 - \text{sensitivity})}{\text{specificity}}$$

Can the results help you?

Is there a SpPIN or SnNOUT?
Can you generate a post-test probability for your patient?
See p. 73.

Is the study valid?

1 Was there a clearly defined question?

What question has the research been designed to answer? Was the question focused in terms of the population group studied, the target disorder and the test(s) considered?

2 Was the presence or absence of the target disorder confirmed with a validated test ('gold' or reference standard)?

How did the investigators know whether or not a patient in the study really had the disease?

To do this, they will have needed some reference standard test (or series of tests) which they know 'always' tells the truth. You need to consider whether the reference standard used is sufficiently accurate.

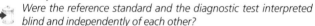

Were the reference standard and the diagnostic test interpreted blind and independently of each other?

If the study investigators know the result of the reference standard test, this might influence their interpretation of the diagnostic test and vice versa.

3 Was the test evaluated on an appropriate spectrum of patients?

A test may perform differently depending upon the sort of patients on whom it is carried out. A test is going to perform better in terms of detecting people with disease if it is used on people in whom the disease is more severe or advanced.

Similarly, the test will produce more false positive results if it is carried out on patients with other diseases that might mimic the disease that is being tested for.

The issue to consider when appraising a paper is whether the test was evaluated on the typical sort of patients on whom the test would be carried out in real life.

4 Was the reference standard applied to all patients?

Ideally, both the test being evaluated and the reference standard should be carried out on all patients in the study. For example, if the test under investigation proves positive, there may be a temptation not to bother administering the reference standard test.

Therefore, when reading the paper you need to find out whether the reference standard was applied to all patients. If it wasn't, look at what steps the investigators took to find out what the 'truth' was in patients who did not have the reference test.

Reference standards

Sometimes, there may not be a single test that is suitable as a reference standard. A range of tests may be needed, and/or an expert panel to decide whether the disease is present or absent. However, this may not be possible for both practical and ethical reasons. For example, the reference test may be invasive and may expose the patient to some risk and/or discomfort.

Is it clear how the test was carried out?
To be able to apply the results of the study to your own clinical practice, you need to be confident that the test is performed in the same way in your setting as it was in the study.

Is the test result reproducible?
This is essentially asking whether you get the same result if different people carry out the test, or if the test is carried out at different times on the same person.

Many studies will assess this by having different observers perform the test, and measuring the agreement between them by means of a kappa statistic. The **kappa** statistic takes into account the amount of agreement that you would expect by chance. If agreement between observers is poor, then the test is not useful.

Kappa

For example, if two observers made a diagnosis by tossing a coin, you would expect them to agree 50% of the time. A kappa score of 0 indicates no more agreement than you would expect by chance; perfect agreement would yield a kappa score of 1. Generally, a kappa score of 0.6 indicates good agreement.

The extent to which the test result is reproducible may depend upon how explicit the guidance is for how the test should be carried out. It may also depend upon the experience and expertise of the observer.

Are the results important?

What is meant by test accuracy?

a The test can correctly detect disease that is present (a true positive result).

b The test can detect disease when it is really absent (a false positive result).

c The test can incorrectly identify someone as being free of a disease when it is present (a false negative result).

d The test can correctly identify that someone does not have a disease (a true negative result).

Ideally, we would like a test which produces a high proportion of a and d and a low proportion of b and c.

Sensitivity and specificity

- **Sensitivity** is the proportion of people with disease who have a positive test.
- **Specificity** is the proportion of people free of a disease who have a negative test.

Sensitivity and specificity

Sensitivity reflects how good the test is at picking up people with disease, while the specificity reflects how good the test is at identifying people without the disease.

These measures are combined into an overall measure of the efficacy of a diagnostic test called the **likelihood ratio**: the likelihood that a given test result would be expected in a patient with the target disorder compared to the likelihood that the same result would be expected in a patient without the disorder).

These possible outcomes of a diagnostic test are illustrated below (sample data from Andriole 1998).

		Target disorder (prostate cancer)		
		Present	**Absent**	**Totals**
Diagnostic test result (prostate serum)	**Positive**	26 **a**	69 **b**	95
	Negative	**c** 46	**d** 249	295
	Totals	72	318	

Sensitivity	a/(a + c)	26/72	= 36%
Specificity	d/(b + d)	249/318	= 78%
Positive predictive value	a/(a + b)	29/95	= 27%
Negative predictive value	d/(c + d)	249/295	= 84%
Pre-test probability (prevalence)	$\frac{(a + c)}{(a + b + c + d)}$	72/390	= 18%
LR for a positive result	$\frac{sens}{(1 - spec)}$	0.36/0.22	= 1.66
LR for a negative result	$\frac{(1 - sens)}{spec}$	0.64/0.78	= 0.82
Pre-test odds	$\frac{Prevalence}{(1 - prevalence)}$	0.18/0.82	= 0.22
For a positive test result:			
Post-test odds	pre-test odds × LR	0.22x1.66	= 0.37
Post-test probability	$\frac{Post\text{-}test\ odds}{(post\text{-}test\ odds + 1)}$	0.37/1.37	= 27%

Using sensitivity and specificity: SpPin and SnNout
Sometimes it can be helpful just knowing the sensitivity and specificity of a test, if they are very high.

If a test has high **specificity**, i.e. if a high proportion of patients without the disorder actually test negative, it is unlikely to produce false positive results. Therefore, if the test is positive it makes the diagnosis very likely.

This can be remembered by the mnemonic **SpPin**: for a test with high specificity (Sp), if the test is positive, then it rules the diagnosis 'in'.

Similarly, with high **sensitivity** a test is unlikely to produce false negative results. This can be remembered by the mnemonic **Sn-Nout**: for a test with high sensitivity (Sn), if the test is negative, then it rules 'out' the diagnosis.

Effect of prevalence

Positive predictive value is the percentage of patients who test positive who actually have the disease. Predictive values are affected by the prevalence of the disease: if a disease is rarer, the positive predictive value will be lower, while sensitivity and specificity are constant.

Since we know that prevalence changes in different health care settings, predictive values are not generally very useful in characterizing the accuracy of tests.

The measure of test accuracy that is most useful when it comes to interpreting test results for individual patients is the **likelihood ratio (LR)**.

Summary

1 Frame the clinical question.
2 Search for evidence concerning the accuracy of the test.
3 Assess the methods used to determine the accuracy of the test.
4 Find out the likelihood ratios for the test.
5 Estimate the pre-test probability of disease in your patient.
6 Apply the likelihood ratios to this pre-test probability using the nomogram to determine what the post-test probability would be for different possible test results.
7 Decide whether or not to perform the test on the basis of your assessment of whether it will influence the care of the patient, and the patient's attitude to different possible outcomes.

Further reading

Altman D. *Practical Statistics for Medical Research*. Edinburgh: Churchill Livingstone, 1991.

Andriole GL, Guess HA, Epstein JI *et al*. Treatment with finasteride preserves usefulness of prostate-specific antigen in the detection of prostate cancer: results of a randomized, double-blind, placebocontrolled clinical trial.

PLESS Study Group. Proscar Long-term Efficacy and Safety Study. *Urology* 1998;**52**(2):195–201. Discussion 201–2.

Fagan TJ. A nomogram for Bayes' Theorem. *N Engl J Med* 1975; **293**:257.

Fleming KA. Evidence-based pathology. *Evidence-Based Medicine* 1997;**2**:132.

Jaeschke R, Guyatt GH, Sackett DL. Users' Guides to the Medical Literature III: How to use an article about a diagnostic test A: Are the results of the study valid? *J Am Med Assoc* 1994;**271**(5):389–91.

Jaeschke R, Guyatt GH, Sackett DL. How to use an article about a diagnostic test A: What are the results and will they help me in caring for my patients? *J Am Med Assoc* 1994;**271**(9):703–7.

Mant J. Studies assessing diagnostic tests. In: Dawes M, Davies P, Gray A, Mant J, Seers K, Snowball R (eds) *Evidence-Based Practice: a primer for health care professionals*. Edinburgh: Churchill Livingstone, 1999, pp. 59–67,133–57.

Richardson WS, Wilson MC, Guyatt GH, Cook DJ, Nishikawa J. How to use an article about disease probability for differential diagnosis. *J Am Med Assoc* 1999;**281**:1214–19.

Sackett DL, Haynes RB, Guyatt GH, Tugwell P. *Clinical Epidemiology; a basic science for clinical medicine*, 2nd edn. Boston: Little, Brown, 1991.

Sackett DL, Straus SE, Richardson WS, Rosenberg WMC, Haynes RB. *Evidence-Based Medicine: How to practice and teach EBM*, 2nd Edn. New York: Churchill Livingstone, 2000.

Nomogram for likelihood ratios

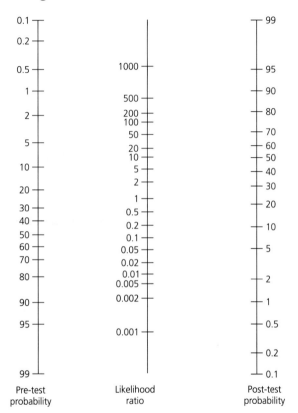

| Pre-test probability | Likelihood ratio | Post-test probability |

How to use the nomogram (Fagan 1975; Sackett 2000)
Position a ruler (or any straight edge) so that it connects the point
on the left hand scale which corresponds to your (estimate of your)
patient's pre-test probability with the point on the middle scale for
the likelihood ratio for their test result. Now read off the post-test
probability on the right-hand scale.

Appraising articles on harm/aetiology

Is the study valid?

1 Was there a clearly defined question?
2 Were there clearly defined, similar groups of patients?
3 Were exposures and clinical outcomes measured the same way in both groups?
4 Was the follow up complete and long enough?
5 Does the suggested causative link make sense?

Are the results important?

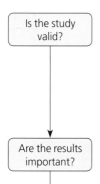

	Adverse outcome	
	Present (case)	Absent (control)
Exposure Positive (cohort)	a	b
Negative (cohort)	c	d

In a randomized controlled trial or cohort study:

$$\text{Relative risk} = \frac{(a\,/\,[a+b])}{(c\,/\,[c+d])}$$

In a case–control study:

$$\text{Odds ratio} = \frac{a \times d}{b \times c}$$

Can the results help you?

Can you calculate an NNH for your PEER? (See p. 74.)

Is the study valid?

In assessing an intervention's potential for harm, we are usually looking at prospective cohort studies or retrospective case–control studies. This is because RCTs may have to be very large indeed to pick up small adverse reactions to treatment.

1 Was there a clearly defined question?

What question has the research been designed to answer? Was the question focused in terms of the population group studied, the exposure received, and the outcomes considered?

2 Were there clearly defined, similar groups of patients?

Studies looking at harm must be able to demonstrate that the two groups of patients are clearly defined and sufficiently similar so as to be comparable. For example, in a cohort study, patients are either exposed to the treatment or not according to a decision. This might mean that sicker patients – perhaps more likely to have adverse outcomes – are more likely to be offered (or demand) potentially helpful treatment. There may be some statistical adjustment to the results to take these potential confounders into account.

3 Were treatment exposures and clinical outcomes measured the same ways in both groups?

You would not want one group to be studied more exhaustively than the other, because this might lead to reporting a greater occurrence of exposure or outcome in the more intensively studied group.

4 Was the follow up complete and long enough?

Follow up has to be long enough for the harmful effects to reveal themselves, and complete enough for the results to be trustworthy (lost patients may have very different outcomes from those who remain in the study).

5 Does the suggested causative link make sense?

You can apply the following rationale to help decide if the results make sense.

- *Is it clear the exposure preceded the onset of the outcome?* It must be clear that the exposure wasn't just a 'marker' of another disease.

- *Is there a dose–response gradient?* If the exposure was causing the outcome, you might expect to see increased harmful effects as a result of increased exposure: a dose–response effect.
- *Is there evidence from a 'dechallenge–rechallenge' study?* Does the adverse effect decrease when the treatment is withdrawn ('dechallenge') and worsen or reappear when the treatment is restarted ('rechallenge')?
- *Is the association consistent from study to study?* Try finding other studies, or, ideally, a systematic review of the question.
- *Does the association make biological sense?* If it does, a causal association is more likely.

Are the results important?

This means looking at the risk or odds of the adverse effect with (as opposed to without) exposure to the treatment; the higher the risk or odds, the stronger the association and the more we should be impressed by it. We can use the single table to determine if the valid results of the study are important.

		Adverse outcome		
		Present (case)	Absent (control)	Totals
Exposure	**Yes (cohort)**	a	b	a+b
	No (cohort)	c	d	b+d
	Totals	a+c	b+d	

In a cohort study:	Relative risk =	$\dfrac{(a/[a+b])}{(c/[c+d])}$
In a case–control study	Odds ratio =	$\dfrac{a \times d}{b \times c}$
To calculate NNH for any OR and PEER		$\dfrac{[PEER (OR - 1)] + 1}{PEER (OR - 1)(1 - PEER)}$

A cohort study compares the risk of an adverse event amongst patients who received the exposure of interest with the risk in a similar group who did not receive it. Therefore, we are able to calculate a relative risk (or risk ratio). In case–control studies, we are presented with the outcomes, and work backwards looking at exposures. Here, we can only compare the two groups in terms of their relative odds (odds ratio).

Statistical significance

As with other measures of efficacy, we would be concerned if the 95% CI around the results, whether relative risk or odds ratio, crossed the value of 1, meaning that there may be no effect (or the opposite).

Further reading

Levine M, Walter S, Lee H, Haines E, Holbrook A, Moyer V, for the Evidence Based Medicine Working Group. Users' Guides to the Medical Literature IV: How to use an article about harm. *J Am Med Assoc* 1994;**272**(20): 1615–19.

Sackett DL, Haynes RB, Guyatt GH, Tugwell P. *Clinical Epidemiology: A basic science for clinical medicine*, 2nd edn. Boston: Little, Brown, 1991.

Sackett DL, Straus SE, Richardson WS, Rosenberg WMC, Haynes RB. *Evidence-Based Medicine: How to practice and teach EBM*, 2nd Edn. New York: Churchill Livingstone, 1996.

Appraising prognosis studies

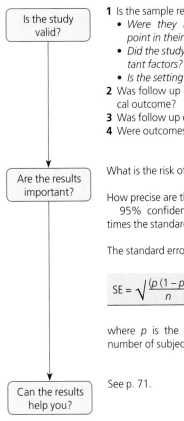

Is the study valid?

1 Is the sample representative?
- *Were they recruited at a common point in their illness?*
- *Did the study account for other important factors?*
- *Is the setting representative?*

2 Was follow up long enough for the clinical outcome?

3 Was follow up complete?

4 Were outcomes measured 'blind'?

Are the results important?

What is the risk of the outcome over time?

How precise are the estimates?

95% confidence intervals are +/–1.96 times the standard error (SE) of a measure.

The standard error for a proportion (*p*) is:

$$SE = \sqrt{\frac{p(1-p)}{n}}$$

where *p* is the proportion and *n* is the number of subjects.

Can the results help you?

See p. 71.

Is the study valid?
In asking questions about a patient's likely prognosis over time, the best individual study type to look for would be longitudinal cohort study.

1 Is the sample representative?
Does the study clearly define the group of patients, and is it similar to your patients? Were there clear inclusion and exclusion criteria?

Were they recruited at a common point in their illness?
The methodology should include a clear description of the stage and timing of the illness being studied. To avoid missing outcomes, study patients should ideally be recruited at an early stage in the disease. In any case, they should all be recruited at a consistent stage in the disease; if not, this will bias the results.

Did the study account for other important factors?
The study groups will have different important variables such as sex, age, weight and co-morbidity which could affect their outcome. The investigators should adjust their analysis to take account of these known factors in different sub-groups of patients. You should use your clinical judgement to assess whether any important factors were left out of this analysis and whether the adjustments were appropriate. This information will also help you in deciding how this evidence applies to your patient.

Is the setting representative?
Patients who are referred to specialist centres often have more illnesses and are higher risk than those cared for in the community. This is sometimes called 'referral bias'.

2 Was follow up long enough for the clinical outcome?
You have to be sure that the study followed the patients for long enough for the outcomes to manifest themselves. Longer follow up may be necessary in chronic diseases.

3 Was follow up complete?
Most studies will lose some patients to follow up; the question you have to answer is whether so many were lost that the information

is of no use to you. You should look carefully in the paper for an account of why patients were lost and consider whether this introduces bias into the result.

- If follow up is less than 80% the study's validity is seriously undermined.

You can ask 'what if' all those patients who were lost to follow up had the outcome you were interested in, and compare this with the study to see if loss to follow up had a significant effect. With low incidence conditions, loss to follow up is more problematic.

4 Were outcomes measured 'blind'?

How did the study investigators tell whether or not the patients actually had the outcome? The investigators should have defined the outcome/s of interest in advance and have clear criteria which they used to determine whether the outcome had occurred. Ideally, these should be objective, but often some degree of interpretation and clinical judgement will be required.

To eliminate potential bias in these situations, judgements should have been applied without knowing the patient's clinical characteristics and prognostic factors.

Are the results important?
What is the risk of the outcome over time?

Three ways in which outcomes might be presented are:

- as a percentage of survival at a particular point in time;
- as a median survival (the length of time by which 50% of study patients have had the outcome);
- as a survival curve that depicts, at each point in time, the proportion (expressed as a percentage) of the original study sample who have not yet had a specified outcome.

Survival curves provide the advantage that you can see how the patient's risk might develop over time.

How precise are the estimates?

Any study looks at a sample of the population, so we would expect some variation between the sample and 'truth'. Prognostic estimates should be accompanied by Confidence Intervals to represent this (see p. 55). You should take account of this range when extracting estimates for your patient. If it is very wide, you would question whether the study had enough patients to provide useful information.

The standard error for a proportion (*p*) is:

$$SE = \sqrt{\frac{p(1-p)}{n}}$$

where *p* is the proportion and *n* is the number of subjects.

Assuming a normal distribution, the 95% confidence interval is 1.96 times this value on either side of the estimate.

Further reading

Laupacis A, Wells G, Richardson WS, Tugwell P. Users' guides to the medical literature. V. How to use an article about prognosis. *J Am Med Assoc* 1994;**272:**234–7.

Sackett DL, Straus SE, Richardson WS, Rosenberg WMC, Haynes RB. *Evidence-Based Medicine: How to practice and teach EBM*, 2nd Edn. New York: Churchill Livingstone, 2000.

Appraising therapy articles

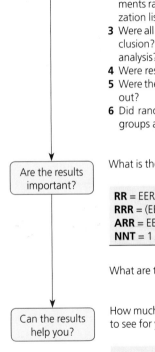

| Is the study valid? | **1** Was there a clearly defined research question? |

1 Was there a clearly defined research question?
2 Was the assignment of patients to treatments randomized and was the randomization list concealed?
3 Were all patients accounted for at its conclusion? Was there an 'intention-to-treat' analysis?
4 Were research participants 'blind'?
5 Were the groups treated equally throughout?
6 Did randomization produce comparable groups at the start of the trial?

Are the results important?

What is the benefit of the treatment?

RR = EER/CER
RRR = (EER − CER) / CER
ARR = EER − CER
NNT = 1 / ARR

What are the confidence intervals?

Can the results help you?

How much of the benefit would you expect to see for your patient?

$$\textbf{NNT} = \frac{1}{((\text{PEER} \times \text{RR}) - \text{PEER})}$$

See p. 74.

Is the study valid?

1 Was there a clearly defined research question?

What question has the research been designed to answer? Was the question focused in terms of the population group studied, the intervention received and the outcomes considered?

2 Were the groups randomized?

The major reason for randomization is to create two (or more) comparison groups which are similar at the start of the trial. To reduce bias as much as possible, the decision as to which treatment a patient receives should be determined by random allocation.

Why is this important?

Randomization is important because it spreads all confounding variables evenly amongst the study groups, even the ones we don't know about.

Jargon

Stratified randomization
Often, there are important clinical features which we already know can affect outcomes. If these are not evenly spread amongst the subjects we could end up with a biased result. Patients can be randomized within these categories to ensure that the that these factors are equally distributed in the control and experimental groups.

Block randomization
Block randomization is a technique for ensuring that each of the treatment groups has the right number of participants while retaining allocation concealment.

Allocation concealment
As a supplementary point, clinicians who are entering patients into a trial may consciously or unconsciously distort the balance between groups if they know the treatments given to previous patients. For this reason, it is preferable that the randomization list be concealed from the clinicians.

This is known as allocation concealment and is the most important thing to look for in appraising RCTs (Schulz 1995).

3 Were all patients accounted for at its conclusion?

There are three major aspects to assessing the follow up of trials:

- Did so many patients drop out of the trial that its results are in doubt?
- Was the study long enough to allow outcomes to become manifest?
- Were patients analysed in the groups to which they were originally assigned?

Intention-to-treat

This means that the patients should *all* be analysed in the groups to which they were originally assigned, even if they switched treatments during the trial.

This is important because it's the only way we can be sure that the original randomization is retained, and therefore that the two groups are comparable.

Drop-out rates

Undertaking a clinical trial is usually time-consuming and difficult to complete properly. If less than 80% of patients are adequately followed up then the results should be ignored.

You look at the follow-up rate reported in the study and ask yourself 'what if everyone who dropped out had a bad outcome?'

Length of study

Studies must allow enough time for outcomes to become manifest. You should use your clinical judgment to decide whether this was true for the study you are appraising, and whether the length of follow up was appropriate to the outcomes you are interested in.

4 Were the research participants 'blinded'?

Ideally, patients and clinicians should not know whether they are receiving the treatment. The assessors may unconsciously bias their assessment of outcomes if they are aware of the treatment. This is known as observer bias.

So, the ideal trial would blind patients, carers, assessors and analysts alike. The terms 'single-', 'double-' and 'triple-blind' are sometimes used to describe these permutations. However, there is some variation in their usage and you should check to see exactly who was blinded in a trial.

Of course, it may have been impossible to blind certain groups of participants, depending on the type of intervention. Researchers should endeavour to get around this, for example by blinding outcomes assessors to the patients' treatment allocation.

Outcome measures

An outcome measure is any feature that is recorded to determine the progression of the disease or problem being studied. Outcomes should be objectively defined and measured wherever possible. Often, outcomes are expressed as mean values of measures rather than numbers of individuals having a particular outcome. The use of means can hide important information about the characteristics of patients who have improved and, perhaps more importantly, those who have got worse.

Note also that concealment of randomization, which happens before patients are enrolled, is different from blinding, which happens afterwards

---

Placebo control

Patients do better if they think they are receiving a treatment than if they do not. A placebo control should be use so that patients can't tell if they're on the active treatment or not.

5 Equal treatment

It should be clear from the article that, for example, there were no co-interventions which were applied to one group but not the other and that the groups were followed similarly with similar check-ups.

6 Did randomization produce comparable groups at the start of the trial?

The purpose of randomization is to generate two (or more) groups of patients who are similar in all important ways. The authors should allow you to check this by displaying important characteristics of the groups in tabular form.

Are the results important?

Two things you need to consider are how large is the treatment effect and how precise is the finding from the trial.

In any clinical therapeutic study there are three explanations for the observed effect:

1 bias;
2 chance variation between the two groups;
3 the effect of the treatment.

Could this result have happened if there was no difference between the groups?

Once bias has been excluded (by asking if the study is valid), we must consider the possibility that the results are a chance effect.

Alongside the results, the paper should report a measure of the likelihood that this result could have occurred if the treatment was no better than the control.

p *values*

The *p* value is a commonly used measure of this probability.

> For example, a *p* value of 0.01 means that there is a 1 in 100 (1%) probability of the result occurring by chance; $p = 0.05$ means this is a 1 in 20 probability.

Conventionally, the value of 0.05 is set as the threshold for statistical significance. If the p value is below 0.05, then the result is statistically significant; it is unlikely to have happened if there was no difference between the groups.

Confidence intervals (CIs)

> Any study can only examine a sample of a population. Hence, we would expect the sample to be different from the population. This is known as *sampling error*. Confidence intervals (CIs) are used to represent sampling error. A 95% CI specifies that there is a 95% chance that the population's 'true' value lies between the two limits.

Look to see if the confidence interval crosses the 'line of no difference' between the interventions. If so, then the result is not statistically significant.

The confidence interval is better than the *p* value because it shows you how much uncertainty there is around the stated result.

Quantifying the risk of benefit and harm

Once chance and bias have been ruled out, we must examine the difference in event rates between the control and experimental groups to see if there is a significant difference. These **event rates** can be calculated as shown below.

	Control	Experimental	Total
Event	a	b	a + b
No Event	c	d	c + d
Total	a+c	b+d	
Event rate	Control event rate CER = a/(a + c)	Experimental event rate EER = b/(b + d)	
Relative risk	EER/CER		
Absolute risk reduction	CER – EER		
Relative risk reduction	$\frac{(CER - EER)}{CER}$		

Relative risk or risk ratio (RR)
RR is the ratio of the risk in the experimental group divided by the risk in the control group.

Absolute risk reduction (ARR)
ARR is the difference between the event rates in the two groups.

Relative risk reduction (RRR)
Relative risk reduction is the ARR as a percentage of the control group risk

RR	ARR	RRR	Meaning
<1	> 0	> 0	Less events in experimental group
1	0	0	No difference between the groups
>1	< 0	< 0	More events in experimental group

ARR is a more clinically relevant measure to use than the RR or RRR. This is because relative measures 'factor out' the baseline risk, so that small differences in risk can seem significant when compared to a small baseline risk.

Number needed to treat (NNT)
Number needed to treat is the most useful measure of benefit, as it tells you the absolute number of patients who need to be treated to prevent one bad outcome. It is the inverse of the ARR:

$$NNT = 1/ARR$$

The confidence interval of an NNT is 1/the CI of its ARR:

$$95\% \text{ CI on the ARR} = \sqrt{\frac{CER(1-CER)}{n\,(control)} + \frac{EER(1-EER)}{n\,(experimental)}}$$

Mortality in patients surviving acute myocardial infarction for at least 3 days with left ventricular ejection fraction <40% (ISIS-4, *Lancet* 1995)		Relative risk reduction (RRR)	Absolute risk reduction (ARR)	Number needed to treat (NNT)
Placebo: control event rate (CER)	Captopril: exp. event rate (EER)	$\dfrac{CER - EER}{CER}$	CER-EER	1/ARR
275/1116 = 0.246	228/1115 = 0.204	(0.246 − 0.204) /0.246 = 17%	0.246 − 0.204 = 0.042	1/0.042 = 24
		(NNTs always round up)		

Summary
An evidence-based approach to deciding whether a treatment is effective for your patient involves the following steps:
1 Frame the clinical question.
2 Search for evidence concerning the efficacy of the therapy.
3 Assess the methods used to carry out the trial of the therapy.
4 Determine the NNT of the therapy.
5 Decide whether the NNT can apply to your patient, and estimate a particularized NNT.
6 Incorporate your patient's values and preferences into deciding on a course of action.

Further reading
Bandolier Guide to Bias: http://www.jr2.ox.ac.uk/bandolier/band80/b80–2.html

Greenhalgh T. *How to Read a Paper*, 3rd edn. Oxford: Blackwell Publishing, 2006.

Guyatt GH, Sackett DL, Cook DJ, for the Evidence Based Medicine Working Group. Users' Guides to the Medical Literature II: How to use an article about therapy or prevention A: Are the results of the study valid? *J Am Med Assoc* 1993;**270**(21):2598–601.

Guyatt GH, Sackett DL, Cook DJ, for the Evidence Based Medicine Working Group. Users' Guides to the Medical Literature II: How to use an article about therapy or prevention B: What were the results and will they help me in caring for my patients? *J Am Med Assoc* 1994:**271**(1):59–63.

ISIS-4 (Fourth International Study of Infarct Survival) Collaborative Group. *Lancet* 1995;**345**:669–85.

Sackett DL, Straus SE, Richardson WS, Rosenberg WMC, Haynes RB. *Evidence-Based Medicine: How to practice and teach EBM*, 2nd Edn. New York: Churchill Livingstone, 2000.

Schulz KF, Chalmers I, Hayes RJ, Altman DG. Empirical evidence of bias: dimensions of methodological quality associated with estimates of treatment effects in controlled trials. *J Am Med Assoc* 1995;**273**:408–12.

Appraising qualitative studies

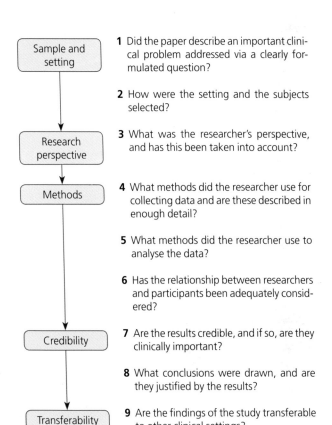

Sample and setting

1 Did the paper describe an important clinical problem addressed via a clearly formulated question?

2 How were the setting and the subjects selected?

Research perspective

3 What was the researcher's perspective, and has this been taken into account?

Methods

4 What methods did the researcher use for collecting data and are these described in enough detail?

5 What methods did the researcher use to analyse the data?

6 Has the relationship between researchers and participants been adequately considered?

Credibility

7 Are the results credible, and if so, are they clinically important?

8 What conclusions were drawn, and are they justified by the results?

Transferability

9 Are the findings of the study transferable to other clinical settings?

Examples of qualitative research methods	
Documents	Study of documentary accounts of events, such as meetings
Passive observation	Systematic watching of behaviour and talk in natural occurring settings
Participant observation	Observation in which the researcher also occupies a role or part in the setting, in addition to observing
Concealed participant observation	The participant observer may be honest about his role in the group, or may conceal the investigation and pretend to be normal member of the group.
In depth interviews	Face to face conversation with the purpose of exploring issues or topics in detail. Does not use preset questions, but is shaped by a defined set of topics
Focus group interviews	Unstructured interviews with small groups of people who interact with each other and the group leader
Consensus method	Used to establish the extent of consensus. There are three main methods: Delphi technique (see p. 23), consensus development panels and nominal group process

Did the paper describe an important clinical problem addressed via a clearly formulated question?

Look for a statement of why the research was done and what specific question it addressed. If not at the outset of the study, by the end of the research process was the research question clear? There is no scientific value in interviewing or observing people just for the sake of it.

You should also consider whether the study used the appropriate design for this question. Would a different method have been more appropriate? For example, if a causal hypothesis was being tested, was a qualitative approach really appropriate?

How were the setting and the subjects selected?

Important questions to consider:
a From where the sample was selected and why?
b Who was selected and why?
c How were they selected and why?

d Was the sample size justified?
e Is it clear why some participants chose not to take part?

Qualitative research usually aims to reflect the diversity within a given population. Research that relies on convenience samples, particularly when the group of interest was difficult to access, will make it difficult to relate the findings to other settings. If you cannot relate your findings to the population you are interested in then you should consider whether it worth continuing.

Purposive (or theoretical) sampling offers researchers a degree of control rather than being at the mercy of any selection bias inherent in pre-existing groups (such as clinic populations). With purposive sampling, researchers deliberately seek to include 'outliers' conventionally discounted in quantitative approaches.

What was the researcher's perspective, and has this been taken into account?

There is no way of abolishing, or fully controlling for, observer bias in qualitative research. This is most obviously the case when participant observation is used, but it is also true for other forms of data collection and of data analysis. Data generated by techniques such as focus groups or semi-structured interviews is likely to be influenced by what the interviewer believes about this subject and by whether he or she is employed by a clinic, the local authority, or a charity group etc. It is inconceivable that the interviews could have been conducted by someone with no views at all and no ideological or cultural perspective. Researchers should therefore describe in detail where they are coming from so that the results can be interpreted accordingly.

What methods did the researcher use for collecting data and are these described in enough detail?

The methods section of a qualitative paper may have to be lengthy since it is telling a unique story without which the results cannot be interpreted. Large amounts of data may be collected. These may include verbatim notes or transcribed recordings of interviews or focus groups, jotted notes and more detailed 'field-notes' of observational research, a diary or chronological account, and the researcher's reflective notes made during the research. The setting is important, for instance patients interviewed in hospital will be biased in their answers as opposed to those interviewed in their homes.

Questions to ask of the data collection are:

1 How the data were collected and why?
2 How the data were recorded and why?
3 If the methods were modified during the process and why?
4 Were the data collected in a way that addresses the research issue?
5 Was their a clear explanation of data saturation

Finally are these methods a sensible and adequate way of addressing the research question.

What methods did the researcher use to analyse the data?

In qualitative research the analytical process begins during data collection as the data already gathered is analysed and shapes the ongoing data collection. This has the advantage of allowing the researcher to go back and refine questions, develop hypotheses, and pursue emerging avenues of inquiry in further depth.

Continuous analysis is inevitable in qualitative research, because the researcher is collecting the data, it is impossible not to start thinking about what is being heard and seen.

Qualitative sampling strategies do not aim to identify a statistically representative set of respondents, so expressing results in relative frequencies may be misleading. Simple counts are sometimes used and may provide a useful summary of some aspects of the analysis.

The researcher must find a systematic way of analysing his or her data, and must seek examples of cases which appear to contradict or challenge the theories derived from the majority. One way of doing this is by content analysis: drawing up a list of coded categories and 'cutting and pasting' each segment of transcribed data into one of these categories. This can be done either manually or via a computer database. Several software packages designed for qualitative data analysis can be used i.e. QSR, NUD.IST and ATLAS.ti.

In theory, the paper will show evidence of quality control: the data (or a sample of them) will have been analysed by more than one researcher to confirm they are both assigning the same meaning to them.

Triangulation addresses the issue of internal validity by using more than one method of data collection to answer a research question. Triangulation compares the results from either two or more different methods of data collection (for example, interviews and observation).

Has the relationship between researchers and participants been adequately considered?

a If the researchers critically examined their role, potential bias and influence?

b Where the data were collected and why that setting was chosen?

c How was the research explained to the participants?

As well as exploration of alternative explanations for the data collected, a long established tactic for improving the quality of explanations in qualitative research is to search for, and discuss, elements in the data that contradict, or seem to contradict, the emerging explanation of the phenomena under study. Such 'deviant case analysis' helps refine the analysis until it can explain all or the vast majority of the cases under scrutiny.

The final technique is to ensure that the research design explicitly incorporates a wide range of different perspectives so that the viewpoint of one group is never presented as if it represents the sole truth about any situation.

Are the results credible, and if so, are they clinically important?

One important aspect of the results section to check is whether the authors cite actual data. The results should be independently and objectively verifiable. A subject either made a particular statement or (s)he did not. All quotes and examples should be indexed so that they can be traced back to an identifiable subject and setting.

What conclusions were drawn, and are they justified by the results?

When assessing the validity of qualitative research, to ask whether the interpretation placed on the data accords with common sense and is relatively untainted with personal or cultural perspective.

a How well does this analysis explain why people behave in the way they do?
b How comprehensible would this explanation be to a thoughtful participant in the setting?
c How well does the explanation cohere with what we already know?

Are the findings of the study transferable to other clinical settings?

One of the commonest criticisms of qualitative research is that the findings of any qualitative study pertain only to the limited setting in which they were obtained. Questions to address are:

a Does the study address the research aim?
b Does the study contribute something new to understanding, new insight or a different perspective?
c What are the inferences for further research?
d What does this study mean in terms of current policy or practice?

How relevant is the research? How important are these findings to practice?

Further reading

Introduction to qualitative methods in health and health services research

Pope and Mays. *Br Med J* 1995;**311**:42–5. http://www.bmj.com/cgi/content/full/311/6996/42

Assessing quality in qualitative research

Mays and Pope. *Br Med J* 2000;**320**:50–2. http://www.bmj.com/cgi/content/full/320/7226/50

Analysing qualitative data

Pope, Ziebland and Mays. *Br Med J* 2000;**320**:114–16. http://www.bmj.com/cgi/content/full/320/7227/114

How to read a paper: papers that go beyond numbers (qualitative research)

Trisha Greenhalgh and Rod Taylor. *Br Med J* 1997;**315**:740–3. http://bmj.bmjjournals.com/cgi/content/full/320/7226/50

Appraising economic evaluations

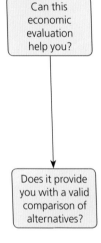

Can this economic evaluation help you?

Does it provide you with a valid comparison of alternatives?

1 Is there good evidence that the interventions are effective?
2 What kind of economic evaluation is it?
   - Cost–consequences study
   - Cost-minimisation study
   - Cost-effectiveness analysis
   - Cost–benefit analysis
   - Cost–utility analysis
3 Is a clear description of the interventions given?
4 Does the economic evaluation address a clearly focused question?

5 Did the study identify all of the relevant costs for each intervention?
6 Did the study include all the relevant outcomes for each intervention?
7 Were costs identified prospectively?
8 What is the perspective of the analysis?
9 Does the evaluation include an appropriate sensitivity analysis?
10 Can the result be applied to the population you are interested in?

Economic evaluations compare the costs and outcomes of two or more treatments or care alternatives.

1 Does the economic evaluation (EE) address a clearly focused question?

Is it clear at the outset what the authors are trying to achieve?

2 What kind of EE is it?

Cost–consequences study:	the outcomes of each intervention are measured in different units, so it's not possible to compare the interventions.
Cost-minimization analysis:	the outcomes are the same for each intervention so we're just interested in which is least costly.
Cost-effectiveness analysis:	the outcomes are different and are measured in natural units, such as blood pressure, event rates or survival rates.
Cost–utility analysis:	the outcomes are different and are measured in patient utilities, such as QALYs.
Cost–benefit analysis:	the outcomes are different and are measured in monetary terms.

3 Is a clear description of the interventions given?

Look for issues of confounding, how complex is the intervention? Is there sufficient information to allow the intervention to be reproduced in clinical practice. Are the interventions feasible?

4 Is there good evidence that the interventions are effective?

This evidence should come from good quality systematic reviews of RCTs, or good quality RCTs. The authors should clearly cite this evidence as the rationale for their economic evaluation.

Does this economic evaluation provide a valid comparison of alternatives?

5 Did the study identify all of the relevant costs for each intervention?

You should be satisfied that the study identified all the relevant costs of delivering the interventions and providing care for their outcomes and valued them credibly. Costs will usually be broken down into two parts:

1 The **unit cost** for each element of an intervention (e.g. cost per GP consultation, cost per hospital day, cost per dose of a drug); and
2 The **resource use**, that is, how many of units of each element were used in the study.

The total cost is the unit cost multiplied by the resource use.

It's important to note that, in comparing different interventions, the analysis should show the costs avoided by providing an intervention that prevents outcomes.

You should consider whether all of the relevant cost elements have been included. For example, costs may be restricted to **direct costs** associate with the intervention (drugs, staff costs in delivering care, costs of providing facilities), and may ignore **indirect costs** such as lost economic productivity, travel costs incurred by patients, etc.

Incremental costs and benefits

Economic evaluations are interested in the **additional** benefits to be gained, and costs incurred, from one intervention as compared to another. This is known as the **incremental** benefits and costs.

---

6 Were costs identified prospectively?

Some (**deterministic**) costs can be predicted in advance, while other (**stochastic**) costs cannot and may vary from one patient to another or from one setting to another. For these reasons, it's best if the evaluation compiles its cost information prospectively during the course of the study rather than retrospectively.

7 Did the study include all the relevant outcomes for each intervention?

Usually, economic evaluations will represent outcomes using natural units (such as number of heart attacks prevented, life-years gained or number of visits to the GP). The disadvantage of such measures is that they don't usually encompass all of the aspects of the intervention.

As noted above, costs for each outcome should be provided so that a cost–benefit analysis can be carried out. The advantage of natural units is that they better reflect clinical priorities.

Sometimes, a cost–utility study will be conducted, in which the possible outcomes are rated by patients using a sliding scale to represent quality of life. This might range from zero (death) to one (perfect health). This helps us to factor in the patients' views into large-scale assessment of cost-effectiveness. Such studies, it's possible to measure the 'amount of health' gained by an intervention rather than just the specific number of events prevented.

QALYs

Quality-Adjusted Life-Years are a **utility** scale. They are a useful measure of outcomes because they combine (objective) survival time with (subjective) patients' quality of life.

Patients are asked to rate a particular state of health on a scale between zero and 1 (where 1 is perfect health and zero is the worst possible state). Often, these are derived with reference to 'Validation studies' that have surveyed a large population and placed a particular value on each specific quality of life.

We can then compare two interventions over time to see how much 'health quality' patients can expect, and therefore how much they might gain (or lose) by adopting a new intervention.

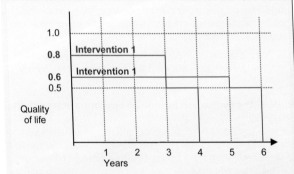

Under Intervention 1, patients can expect 3 years at a Quality of Life (QoL) of 0.8 plus one year at 0.5. This equates to $((3 \times 0.8) + (1 \times 0.5)) = 2.9$ QALYs.

Intervention 2 gives 5 years at 0.6 QALYs plus one year at 0.5, or $((5 \times 0.6) + (1 \times 0.5)) = 3.5$ QALYs.

So Intervention 2 gives patients 0.6 QALYs more than Intervention 1.

8 What is the perspective of the analysis?

The evaluation should state the perspective from which it was carried out. Costs and benefits may be different from a patient's perspective than from a health care provider's. For example, creating a primary care 'drop-in' centre may increase costs from the perspective of the health care provider, but could reduce costs from the perspective of individuals, employers and society as a whole by making it easier for people to access services without taking time off work.

Can an analysis from this perspective help you to answer your question?

Discounting

Economists use discounting to account for the fact that a cost or benefit we get now is worth more than the same benefit in the future. It is standard practice to discount costs at 6% per year and benefits at 1.5% per year.

This means that if a drug costs £1000 per year over two years, its cost in year 2 is (1000 − 6% =) £940 when evaluated in year one.

---

9 Does the evaluation include an appropriate sensitivity analysis?

Because costs and benefits can be different in different settings and at different times, the study should report a sensitivity analysis to show how much the findings would be affected by changes in the cost or benefit data.

So, for example, increases in the price of drugs or in the cost of delivering a service might reduce the overall cost-effectiveness of a new intervention.

10 Can the result be applied to the population you are interested in?

The main points to consider here are: the similarity of the patients in the review to the population you are interested in. Can you afford the intervention, will the money have to come from another service to fund the intervention. Do you have the resources or the personnel to deliver a new service?

Applying the evidence

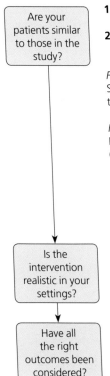

Are your patients similar to those in the study?

1 Are they so different that the results can't help you?
2 How much of the study effect can you expect for your patients?

For diagnostic tests
Start with your patient's pre-test probability then use the nomogram on page 41.

For therapy
Estimate your patient's expected event rate (PEER):

$$\textbf{NNT} = \frac{1}{(\text{PEER} \times \text{RRR})}$$

Is the intervention realistic in your settings?

3 Is the intervention realistic in your setting?
4 Does the comparison intervention reflect your current practice?
5 What alternatives are available?

Have all the right outcomes been considered?

6 Are the outcomes appropriate to your patient?
7 Does the intervention meet their values and preferences?

Are your patients similar to those of the study?

Of course, your patients weren't in the trial, so you need to apply your clinical expertise to decide whether they are sufficiently similar for the results to be applicable to them. Factors which would affect this decision include:

- The age range included in the trial (many trials exclude the older generations); your group of patients may have a different risk profile. For example, although many drugs have increasing adverse effects in the ageing population which may not be taken into account in the study, they may also have greater benefits.
- Many of your patients will have co-morbidity which could affect drug interactions and adverse events as well as benefits.
- Will your patients be able to comply with treatment dosages and duration? For example, compliance might decrease if your patient is taking other medications or if the treatment requires multiple doses daily rather than single ones.
- If NNTs are similar for different treatments, then the NNHs for harmful side effects will become more important; lesser side effects may increase compliance (Bloom, 2001).

The inclusion and exclusion criteria for the study may help as a starting point for your clinical judgment here. It is unlikely, however, that your patient will present an exact match with the study; Sackett *et al* (2000) have recommended framing this question in reverse:

How different would your patient have to be for the results of the study to be of no help?

How much of the study effect can you expect for your patient(s)?

To work out how much effect your patient can expect from the intervention, you first need an estimate of their risk of the outcome. This information might be available from a number of external sources, such as cardiovascular risk tables in the British National Formulary, systematic reviews, Department of Health data or even local audit data.

The control group in the study may also provide a good starting point. However, you should use your clinical judgment to arrive at an individual's risk, taking account of his or her individual clinical characteristics.

Diagnosis

In diagnostic tests, you need to derive an estimate of your patients' pre-test probability, that is the likelihood that they have the disorder prior to doing the test. The prevalence from the study population may act as a guide. Trial data may exist which it generates sensitivities, specificities and LRs for clinical symptoms and signs; see the Rational Clinical Examination series in the *Journal of the American Medical Association*, 1992–2001. This can be combined with the likelihood ratio of the test result to generate a post-test probability.

> The term **prevalence** is applied to populations; **pre-test probability** is applied to individuals.

To calculate a post-test probability, you first need to convert your pre-test probability into pre-test odds (see Altman 1991 for more details):

$$\text{Pre-test odds} = \frac{\text{pre-test probability}}{(1 - \text{pre-test probability})}$$

You can now multiply by the test result's likelihood ratio to yield the post-test odds:

$$\text{Post-test odds} = \text{pre-test odds} \times \text{LR}$$

In turn, these post-test odds can be converted back into a post-test probability:

$$\text{Post-test probability} = \frac{\text{post-test odds}}{(\text{post-test odds} + 1)}$$

However, in the interests of simplicity, we suggest you either use the nomogram on page 41 or the diagnostic calculator at http://www.cebm.net.

The post-test probability from one test can be used as the pre-test probability for the next in a series of independent tests.

Once you have a set of LRs, sensitivities and specificities of the tests you perform, you will quickly see that your post-test probabilities are very much influenced by pretest probabilities. In the acute setting your clinical judgment will largely determine your patient's pre-test probability.

You will see that, for low, intermediate and high probabilities, tests vary widely in their usefulness.

Therapy
Two ways of estimating an individual patient's benefit have been suggested by Sackett *et al* (2000).

f Method
This requires that you estimate your patient's risk compared to the control group from the study. Thus, if your patient is twice as susceptible as those in the trial, $f = 2$; if half as susceptible, $f = 0.5$. Assuming the treatment produces the same relative risk reduction for patients at different levels of risk, the NNT for your patient is simply the trials reported NNT divided by f.

$$\text{NNT (for your patient)} = \frac{\text{NNT}}{f}$$

Note, however, that if the NNT's confidence intervals are close to the line of no difference, this method becomes less reliable, as it will not detect the point at which those CIs cross the line.

Patient Expected Event Rate (PEER) Method
Alternatively, you could start from an estimate of your patient's risk of an event (expected event rate) without the treatment. This estimate could be based on the study's control group or other prognostic evidence, but you should use your clinical judgment.

Multiply this PEER by the RRR for the study: the result is your patient's ARR, which can be inverted to yield the NNT for your patient.

$$\text{NNT (for your patient)} = \frac{1}{(\text{PEER} \times \text{RRR})}$$

We assume that the same relative benefit would apply to patients at different levels of risk.

Is the intervention realistic in your setting?

You need to consider whether the treatment, test, prognostic factor or causative described in the study would be comparable in your setting, and to what extent any differences would affect your judgement. Amongst the factors you should consider are:

- Did the study take place in a different country, with different demographics?
- Did it take place in a different clinical setting (in-patient, district general, teaching hospital, emergency department, out-patient, general practice)?
- Some interventions, especially diagnostic tests, may be unavailable or slow to come back.
- Will you be able to provide a comparable level of monitoring?
- How you present the treatment options to the patient will be different from the trial; this might significantly affect patient compliance.

Does the comparison intervention reflect your current practice?

If the study compares the benefits of new intervention A with control intervention B, does B match up with what you currently do? If not, you need to think about how your current practice would compare and whether this would affect the extent of any benefit.

Translating an intervention to your practice setting may open up a whole gamut of issues, which we can only touch upon here. However, it is worth asking whether you can adapt your setting. For instance:

- Can your practice nurse develop specialist clinics?
- Can one of your GPs develop a specialist interest?
- Can you introduce protocols which are evidence-based which can be followed by a number of staff, irrespective of seniority?
- Can your guidelines be transferable between different wards or settings?

- How can you maximize your time to make sure that your intervention is realistic in your setting?
- Do your staff need extra training?
- Do you need to do a cost–benefit analysis?
- Are you going to audit what you do? Do you need to follow up your patients?

What alternatives are available?

There may be different ways of tackling the same disorder, such as in hypertension, where evidence may be for single or combined drug effects. Again, dosage and delivery are likely to affect compliance, which in turn may make alternatives more practical.

- Have you weighed up the adverse effects of your treatment against those of less helpful treatments? You (or your patient) may feel that a treatment of less benefit which is less harmful may be more appropriate.
- Is doing nothing an option? This relies on your interpretation of the patient's benefits and risk of harm, and what the patient thinks.
- Is there a class effect? Many trials put down the effect to the specific drug and not the generic class.
- Is your patient on so many drugs that it might be worth stopping some or all of them if the adverse effects outweigh the benefits?
- Is your patient aware of lifestyle changes which may be of benefit?

Are the outcomes appropriate to your patient?

What does your patient think? Does your patient understand the implications of the intervention? Some drugs require lifelong adherence to maintain efficacy. The outcomes which are important to you are not necessarily the ones which matter most to your patient, particularly where quality of life is affected. Other important issues to discuss with your patient include:

- Some of the adverse effects may not be mentioned in trials, but may be very relevant to your patient, such as mood disturbances.
- How much reassurance would your patient derive from test results or prognostic estimates?
- The invasiveness of a test or procedure may affect your patient's willingness to participate.
- Implications for further testing and/or treatment.

Further reading

Altman D. *Practical Statistics for Medical Research*. Edinburgh: Churchill Livingstone, 1991.

Bloom BS. Daily regimen and compliance with treatment. *Br Med J* 2001;**323**:647.

Sackett DL, Straus SE, Richardson WS, Rosenberg WMC, Haynes RB. *Evidence-Based Medicine: How to practice and teach EBM*, 2nd Edn. New York: Churchill Livingstone, 2000.

Evidence-based medicine: glossary of terms

http://www.cebm.net

Absolute risk reduction (ARR): the difference in the event rate between control group (CER) and treated group (EER): ARR = CER − EER. *See p. 55.*

Adjustment: a summarizing procedure for a statistical measure in which the effects of differences in composition of the populations being compared have been minimized by statistical methods.

All or none: a treatment benefit where, previously, all patients died but now some survive, or previously some patients died but now all survive.

Association: statistical dependence between two or more events, characteristics, or other variables. An association may be fortuitous or may be produced by various other circumstances; the presence of an association does not necessarily imply a causal relationship.

Bias: any tendency to influence the results of a trial (or their interpretation) other than the experimental intervention.

Blinding: a technique used in research to eliminate bias by hiding the intervention from the patient, clinician, and/or other researchers who are interpreting results.

Blind(ed) study (masked study): A study in which observer(s) and/or subjects are kept ignorant of the group to which the subjects are assigned, as in an experimental study, or of the population from which the subjects come, as in a non-experimental or observational study.

Blobbogram: *see* Forrest plot.

Case–control study: involves identifying patients who have the outcome of interest (cases) and control patients without the same outcome, and looking to see if they had the exposure of interest.

Case-series: a report on a series of patients with an outcome of interest. No control group is involved.

CER: control event rate; *see* Event rate.

Clinical practice guideline: a systematically developed statement designed to assist health care professionals and patients make decisions about appropriate health care for specific clinical circumstances.

Cochrane collaboration: a worldwide association of groups who create and maintain systematic reviews of the literature for specific topic areas.

Coding: the assignment of (usually numeric) codes to each category of each variable.

Cohort study: involves the identification of two groups (cohorts) of patients, one which did receive the exposure of interest, and one which did not, and following these cohorts forward for the outcome of interest.

Co-interventions: interventions other than the treatment under study that are applied differently to the treatment and control groups. Co-intervention is a serious problem when double blinding is absent or when the use of very effective non-study treatments is permitted.

Co-morbidity: co-existence of a disease or diseases in a study participant in addition to the index condition that is the subject of study.

Comparison group: any group to which the intervention group is compared. Usually synonymous with control group.

Confidence interval (CI): the range around a study's result within which we would expect the true value to lie. CIs account for the sampling error between the study population and the wider population the study is supposed to represent. *See p. 55.*

Confounding variable: a variable which is not the one you are interested in but which may affect the results of trial.

Content analysis: the systematic analysis of observations obtained from records, documents and field notes.

Cost–benefit analysis: converts effects into the same monetary terms as the costs and compares them.

Cost-effectiveness analysis: converts effects into health terms and describes the costs for some additional health gain (for example, cost per additional MI prevented).

Cost–utility analysis: converts effects into personal preferences (or utilities) and describes how much it costs for some additional quality gain (e.g. cost per additional quality-adjusted life-year, or QUALY).

Critically appraised topic (CAT): a short summary of an article from the literature, created to answer a specific clinical question.

Crossover study design: the administration of two or more experimental therapies one after the other in a specified or random order to the same group of patients.

Cross-sectional study: a study that observes a defined population at a single point in time or time interval. Exposure and outcome are determined simultaneously.

Decision analysis: the application of explicit, quantitative methods to analyse decisions under conditions of uncertainty.

Determinant: any definable factor that effects a change in a health condition or other characteristic.

Dose–response relationship: a relationship in which change in amount, intensity, or duration of exposure is associated with a change – either an increase or decrease – in risk of a specified outcome.

Ecological survey: a study based on aggregated data for some population as it exists at some point or points in time; to investigate the relationship of an exposure to a known or presumed risk factor for a specified outcome.

EER: experimental event rate; *see* Event rate.

Effectiveness: a measure of the benefit resulting from an intervention for a given health problem under usual conditions of clinical care for a particular group.

Efficacy: a measure of the benefit resulting from an intervention for a given health problem under the ideal conditions of an investigation.

Ethnography: the study of people in their natural settings; a descriptive account of social life and culture in a defined social system, based on qualitative methods.

Event rate: the proportion of patients in a group in whom an event is observed. *See p. 55.*

Evidence-based health care: the application of the principles of evidence-based medicine (see below) to all professions associated with health care, including purchasing and management.

Evidence-based medicine: the conscientious, explicit, and judicious use of current best evidence in making decisions about the care of individual patients. The practice of evidence-based medicine means integrating individual clinical expertise with the best available external clinical evidence from systematic research.

Exclusion criteria: conditions that preclude entrance of candidates into an investigation even if they meet the inclusion criteria.

f: an estimate of the chance of an event for your patient, expressed as a decimal fraction of the control group's risk (event rate). *See p. 74.*

Focus groups: a research method of interviewing people while they are interacting in small groups.

Follow up: observation over a period of time of an individual, group, or initially defined population whose relevant characteristics have been assessed in order to observe changes in health status or health-related variables.

Forrest plot: a diagrammatic representation of the results of individual trials in a meta-analysis.

Funnel plot: a method of graphing the results of trials in a meta-analysis to show if the results have been affected by publication bias.

Gold standard: *see* Reference standard.

Grounded theory: an approach to qualitative research in which the investigator develops conceptual categories from the data and then makes new observations to develop these categories. Hypotheses are developed directly form data.

Heterogeneity: in systematic reviews, the amount of incompatibility between trials included in the review, whether clinical (i.e. the studies are clinically different) or statistical (i.e. the results are different from one another).

Incidence: the number of new cases of illness commencing, or of persons falling ill, during a specified time period in a given population.

Intention-to-treat: characteristic of a study where patients are analysed in the groups to which they were originally assigned, even though they may have switched treatment arms during the study for clinical reasons.

Interviewer bias: systematic error due to interviewer's subconscious or conscious gathering of selective data.

Lead-time bias: if prognosis study patients are not all enrolled at similar, welldefined points in the course of their disease, differences in outcome over time may merely reflect differences in duration of illness.

Likelihood ratio: the likelihood that a given test result would be expected in a patient with the target disorder compared to the likelihood that the same result would be expected in a patient without that disorder. *See pp. 37–41.*

MeSH: medical subject headings: a thesaurus of medical terms used by many databases and libraries to index and classify medical information.

Meta-analysis: a systematic review which uses quantitative methods to summarize the results.

N-of-1 trial: the patient undergoes pairs of treatment periods organized so that one period involves the use of the experimental treatment and one period involves the use of an alternate or placebo therapy. The patients and physician are blinded, if possible, and outcomes are monitored. Treatment periods are replicated until the clinician and patient are convinced that the treatments are definitely different or definitely not different.

Naturalistic research: descriptive research in natural, un-manipulated social settings using unobtrusive qualitative methods.

Negative predictive value (−PV): the proportion of people with a negative test who are free of disease.

Neyman bias: bias due to cases being missed because they have not had time to develop or are too mild to be detected at the time of the study.

Number needed to treat (NNT): the number of patients who need to be treated to prevent one bad outcome. It is the inverse of the ARR: NNT = 1/ARR. *See p. 56.*

Observer bias: bias in a trial where the measurement of outcomes or disease severity may be subject to bias because observers are not blinded to the patients' treatment.

Odds: a ratio of events to non-events. If the event rate for a disease is 0.1 (10%), its non-event rate is 0.9 and therefore its odds are 1/9.

Outcomes research: evaluates the impact of health care on the health outcomes of patients and populations.

Overview: a summary of medical literature in a particular area.

***p* value:** the probability that a particular result would have happened by chance.

PEER: patient expected event rate: an estimate of the risk of an outcome for your patient.

Phenomenology: an approach to qualitative research which concerns itself with the study of individual experiences.

Placebo: an inactive version of the active treatment that is administered to patients.

Positive predictive value (+PV): the proportion of people with a positive test who have disease.

Post-test probability: the probability that a patient has the disorder of interest after the test result is known.

Pre-test probability: the probability that a patient has the disorder of interest prior to administering a test.

Prevalence: the baseline risk of a disorder in the population of interest.

Prospective study: study design where one or more groups (**cohorts**) of individuals who have not yet had the outcome event in question are monitored for the number of such events which occur over time.

Publication bias: a bias in a systematic review caused by incompleteness of the search, such as omitting non-English language sources, or unpublished trials (inconclusive trials are less likely to be published than conclusive ones, but are not necessarily less valid).

Randomized controlled clinical trial: a group of patients is randomized into an experimental group and a control group. These groups are followed up for the variables/outcomes of interest.

Recall bias: systematic error due to the differences in accuracy or completeness of recall to memory of past events or experiences.

Reference standard: a diagnostic test used in trials to confirm presence or absence of the target disorder.

Referral filter bias: the sequence of referrals that may lead patients from primary to tertiary centres raises the proportion of more severe or unusual cases, thus increasing the likelihood of adverse or unfavourable outcomes.

Relative risk (RR) (or risk ratio): the ratio of the risk of an event in the experimental group compared to that of the control group (RR = EER/CER). Not to be confused with relative risk reduction (see below). *See p. 56.*

Relative risk reduction (RRR): the percentage reduction in events in the treated group event rate (EER) compared to the control group event rate (CER): RRR = (CER − EER)/CER. *See p. 55.*

Reproducibility (repeatability, reliability): the results of a test or measure are identical or closely similar each time it is conducted.

Retrospective study: study design in which cases where individuals who had an outcome event in question are collected and analysed after the outcomes have occurred.

Risk: the probability that an event will occur for a particular patient or group of patients. Risk can be expressed as a decimal fraction or percentage (0.25 = 25%).

Risk ratio: *see* Relative risk.

Selection bias: a bias in assignment or selection of patients for a study that arises from study design rather than by chance. This can occur when the study and control groups are chosen so that they differ from each other by one or more factors that may affect the outcome of the study.

Sensitivity: the proportion of people with disease who have a positive test.

Sensitivity analysis: a process of testing how sensitive a result would be to changes in factors such as baseline risk, susceptibility, the patients' best and worst outcomes, etc.

SnNout: when a sign/test has a high sensitivity, a negative result rules out the diagnosis.

Specificity: the proportion of people free of a disease who have a negative test.

Spectrum bias: a bias caused by a study population whose disease profile does not reflect that of the intended population (for example, if they have more severe forms of the disorder).

SpPin: when a sign/test has a high specificity, a positive result rules in the diagnosis.

Stratification: division into groups. Stratification may also refer to a process to control for differences in confounding variables, by making separate estimates for groups of individuals who have the same values for the confounding variable.

Strength of inference: the likelihood that an observed difference between groups within a study represents a real difference rather than mere chance or the influence of confounding factors, based on both p values and confidence intervals. Strength of inference is weakened by various forms of bias and by small sample sizes.

Survival curve: a graph of the number of events occurring over time or the chance of being free of these events over time. The events must be discrete and the time at which they occur must be precisely known. In most clinical situations, the chance of an outcome changes with time. In most survival curves the earlier follow up periods usually include results from more patients than the later periods and are therefore more precise.

Systematic review: an article in which the authors have systematically searched for, appraised, and summarized all of the medical literature for a specific topic.

Validity: the extent to which a variable or intervention measures what it is supposed to measure or accomplishes what it is supposed to accomplish. The **internal validity** of a study refers to the integrity of the experimental design. The **external validity** of a study refers to the appropriateness by which its results can be applied to non-study patients or populations.

Selected evidence-based healthcare resources on the web

For a live list of these links, go to:
http://www.minervation.com/EBMtoolkit/EBMlinks.html

Abstracts of Cochrane Reviews
http://www.cochrane.org/cochrane/revabstr/mainindex.htm
Alphabetical list of Cochrane reviews.

Allied and Complementary Medicine Database (AMED)
http://edina.ac.uk/cab
AMED is an abstract database produced by the Health Care Information Service of the British Library. It covers a selection of journals in three separate subject areas; allied to medicine, complementary medicine and palliative care. Numerous of the 512 journals included are not indexed elsewhere.

American College of Physicians
http://www.acponline.org/

ACP journal club
http://www.acpjc.org/?hp
Online version of the ACP journal.

Appraisal of Guidelines Research and Evaluation AGREE
http://www.agreecollaboration.org/
AGREE stands for 'Appraisal of Guidelines Research and Evaluation'. It originates from an international collaboration of researchers and policy makers who work together to improve the quality and effectiveness of clinical practice guidelines by establishing a shared framework for their development, reporting and assessment.

Bandolier
http://www.jr2.ox.ac.uk/bandolier

Best Evidence
http://ebm.bmjjournals.com

BIOME
http://biome.ac.uk/
Barrier free access to peer reviewed research.

CATBank: University of Michigan
http://www.med.umich.edu/pediatrics/ebm/Cat.htm
Department of paediatrics CatBank.

CATBank: BestBETs
http://www.bestbets.org/
BETs were developed in the Emergency Department of Manchester Royal Infirmary, UK, to provide rapid evidence-based answers to real-life clinical questions, using a systematic approach to reviewing the literature. BETs take into account the shortcomings of much current evidence, allowing physicians to make the best of what there is.

CAT Crawler
http://www.bii.a-star.edu.sg/research/mig/cat_search.asp
Search engine for a number of CAT sites on the net.

Centre for Evidence Based Medicine
http://www.cebm.net
Centre for EBM based in Oxford with information on courses, tips, downloads, accessible power point presentations to download and more.

Centre for Evidence Based Child Health
http://www.ich.ucl.ac.uk/ich/academicunits/Centre_for_
evidence_based_child_health/
The Centre for Evidence-Based Child Health was established by Great Ormond Street Hospital Trust and the Institute of Child Health, London, in 1995 as a part of a national network of Centres for Evidence-Based Health Care. The centre's activities build on the experience and expertise of the Centre for Paediatric Epidemiology and Biostatistics and on the clinical links with Great Ormond Street Hospital.

Centre for Evidence-Based Medicine, Mount Sinai, Toronto, including packages on practising EBM
http://www.cebm.utoronto.ca/
The goal of this website is to help develop, disseminate, and evaluate resources that can be used to practise and teach EBM for undergraduate, postgraduate and continuing education for health care professionals from a variety of clinical disciplines.

Centre for Evidence-Based Mental Health in Oxford
http://www.cebmh.com/
Promoting and supporting the teaching and practice of evidence-based mental healthcare.

Centre for Evidence-Based Nursing in York
http://www.york.ac.uk/healthsciences/centres/evidence/cebn.htm
The Centre for Evidence-Based Nursing CEBN) is concerned with furthering EBN through education, research and development.

Centre for Evidence-Based Social Services in Exeter
http://www.cebss.org/
A partnership between The Department of Health, a consortium of Social Services Departments in the South West of England and the University of Exeter (Peninsula Medical School). The main aim is to ensure that decisions taken at all levels in Social Services are informed by trends from good-quality research.

Centres for Health Evidence
http://www.cche.net/che/home.asp
Based in Canada, where they have loads of EBH resources, including critical appraisal worksheets and the JAMA Guides.

Clinical Evidence
http://www.clinicalevidence.org

Cochrane Library
http://www.thecochranelibrary.com

The international Cochrane Collaboration homepage
http://www.cochrane.org

COPAC
http://copac.ac.uk/
Provides free access to the online catalogues of the British Library, National Library of Scotland and 23 university research libraries in the UK and Ireland, covering the full range of health and life science subjects.

DISCERN
http://www.discern.org.uk/
A tool to evaluate clinical information publications, directed primarily to consumers of health care.

Duke University Medical Center Library and Health Sciences Library
http://www.hsl.unc.edu/services/tutorials/ebm/welcome.htm
Tutorials on evidence-based practice for any health care practitioner or student who needs a basic introduction to the principles of evidence-based medicine.

EBM Online
http://ebm.bmjjournals.com/
Evidence-based medicine surveys a wide range of international medical journals applying strict criteria for the quality and validity of research. Practising clinicians assess the clinical relevance of the best studies. The key details of these essential studies are presented in a succinct, informative abstract with an expert commentary on its clinical application.

Electronic Statistics Textbook
http://www.statsoft.com/textbook/stathome.html
This Electronic Statistics Textbook offers training in the understanding and application of statistics.

EPIQ: Effective Practice, Informatics and Quality Improvement
http://www.health.auckland.ac.nz/population-health/epidemiology-biostats/epiq/
Tools and resources for putting it all into practice, including Rod Jackson's GATE tool.

Evidence Based Health Care
http://www.uic.edu/depts/lib/lhsp/resources/ebm.shtml
The guide is designed to assist health care professionals and students become effective and efficient users of the medical literature, provided by the University of Illinois Chicago.

Evidence Based Medicine Tools
http://pedsccm.wustl.edu/EBJ/EBM_Tools_ReadMe.html
A Microsoft Word 97/98 template file that performs numerous clinical epidemiology calculations, e.g., relative risk reduction, likelihood ratios, etc., and the relevant confidence intervals.

Evidence Based Medicine Resource Center
http://www.ebmny.org/
Resource centre from the New York Academy of Medicine.

HIRU – The Health Informatics Research Unit
http://hiru.mcmaster.ca/
Based at McMaster University's Department of Clinical Epidemiology and Biostatistics in Canada, features a large inventory of evidence-based resources and an on-line database.

InfoPOEMS
http://www.infopoems.com/
CAT-style Patient-Oriented Evidence that Matters.

Library for Evidence Based Practice available on the web
http://www.shef.ac.uk/scharr/ir/core.html
A virtual library that has been put together by assembling links to full-text documents on all aspects of evidence-based practice.

Masters in Evidence-Based Health Care Oxford
http://www.conted.ox.ac.uk/cpd/healthsciences/
Oxford University's Department for Continuing Education offer a part-time course in evidence-based health care.

MEDLINE (PubMed)
http://www.pubmed.gov

National Library for Health (NeLH)
http://www.library.nhs.uk

National Guideline Clearinghouse
http://www.guideline.gov/

Primary Care Clinical Practice Guidelines
http://medicine.ucsf.edu/resources/guidelines/
Compiled by Peter Sam, University of California School of Medicine.

Resources for Practising EBM
http://pedsccm.wustl.edu/EBJ/EB
A comprehensive and concise bibliography of evidence-based medicine resources.

SALSER
http://edina.ed.ac.uk/salser/
A catalogue of serials holdings in all Scottish universities.

On-line Public Access Catalogues (OPACs): ScHARR Introduction to Evidence Based Practice on the Internet
http://www.shef.ac.uk/scharr/ir/netting/A
Netting the Evidence is intended to facilitate evidence-based healthcare by providing support and access to helpful organizations and useful learning resources, such as an evidence-based virtual library, software and journals.

SIGN (Scottish Intercollegiate Guidelines Network)
http://www.sign.ac.uk/methodology/filters.html
Validated search strategies for finding high-quality evidence.

Statistical calculators
http://members.aol.com/johnp71/javastat.html
A powerful, conveniently accessible, multi-platform statistical software package. There are also links to online statistics books, tutorials, download-able software, and related resources.
http://www.med.utah.edu/pem/calculators/
Spreadsheets in Excel to calculate odds ratios, confidence intervals, sample size estimates, etc.

SUMsearch
http://sumsearch.uthscsa.edu/searchform45.htm

The NHS Centre for Reviews and Dissemination at York
http://www.york.ac.uk/inst/crd/
CRD undertakes reviews of research about the effects of interventions used in health and social care. The centre maintains various databases provides an enquiry service and disseminates results of research to NHS decision makers.

The PedsCCM Evidence-Based Journal Club
http://pedsccm.wustl.edu/EBJournal_club.html
A journal club for paediatric critical care.

TRIP database
http://www.tripdatabase.com

University of Alberta
http://www.med.ualberta.ca/ebm/ebmtoc.htm
Sources of evidence.

University of British Columbia Clinical Significance Calculator
http://www.healthcare.ubc.ca/calc/clinsig.html
Contingency table analysis to determine risks and odds ratios and their 95% confidence intervals.

ZETOC: British Library electronic table of contents
http://zetoc.mimas.ac.uk
A searchable database of approx 22 million articles covering every field of academic study. Copies of articles and conference papers listed on the database can be ordered online from the British Library's Document Supply Centre.

Non-English language evidence-based healthcare sites

Critique et Pratique
http://machaon.fmed.ulaval.ca/medecine/cetp/
A journal club in French run by Laval University Family Medicine Department.

Stiftung Paracelsus heute in Switzerland
http://www.paracelsus-heute.ch/
Critical appraisal of diagnostic, therapeutic and preventive interventions of modern as well as unconventional medicine, plus courses, symposia and research using EBM techniques.

Evidence-Based Medicine in Switzerland
http://www.evimed.ch/
A journal club and EBM site in German.

Ulmer Initiative für Evidence-Based Medicine
http://www.uni-ulm.de/cebm/

IAMBE
http://www.iambe.org.ar/
Instituto Argentino de Medicina Basada en las Evidencias, in Spanish.

CASP Espana
http://www.redcaspe.org/
Critical Appraisal Skills Programme, in Spanish.

Gruppo Italiano per la Medicina Basata sulle Evidenze (GIMBE)
http://www.gimbe.org/
Evidence-based medicine Italian group.

Evidence-Based Medicine in Taiwan
http://www.cch.org.tw/ebm
An introduction to evidence-based medicine in Chinese (set up
your browser to accept Chinese characters!).

Evidence-Based Medicine
http://www.med.nihon-u.ac.jp/department/public_
health/ebm/
In Japanese, based at the Department of Public Health of the
University of Nihon.

Moscow Centre for EBM and Pharmacotherapy
http://evbmed.fbm.msu.ru/
Providing support for evidence-based health care in Russian.

Levels of evidence

Level	Rx/prevention, aetiology/harm	Prognosis	Diagnosis	Economic analysis
1a	SR[1] of RCTs	SR of inception cohort studies; or a validated CPG[2]	SR of Level 1 diagnostic studies; or a CPG validated on a test set	SR of Level 1 economic studies
1b	Individual RCT (with narrow Confidence interval)	Individual inception cohort study with ≥ 80% follow up	Independent blind comparison of patients from an appropriate spectrum of patients, all of whom have undergone both the diagnostic test and the reference standard	Analysis comparing alternative outcomes against appropriate cost measurement, including a sensitivity analysis
1c	all or none	All or none case-series	Absolute SpPins and SnNouts	Clearly as good or better, but cheaper. Clearly as bad or worse but more expensive. Clearly better or worse at the same cost
2a	SR of cohort studies	SR of either retrospective cohort studies or untreated control groups in RCTs	SR of Level ≥2 diagnostic studies	SR of Level ≥2 economic studies

Level	Rx/prevention, aetiology/harm	Prognosis	Diagnosis	Economic analysis
2b	Individual cohort study (including low quality RCT; e.g. <80% follow up)	Retrospective cohort study or follow-up of untreated control patients in an RCT; or CPG not validated in a test set	Any of: • Independent blind or objective comparison; • Study performed in a set of non-consecutive patients, or confined to a narrow spectrum of study individuals (or both) all of whom have undergone both the test and the reference standard; • A diagnostic CPG not validated in a test set	Analysis comparing a limited number of alternative outcomes against appropriate cost measurement, and including a sensitivity analysis incorporating clinically sensible variations in important variables
2c	'Outcomes' Research	'Outcomes' Research		
3a	SR of case–control studies			
3b	Individual case–control Study		Independent blind or objective comparison of an appropriate spectrum but the reference standard was not applied to all study patients	Analysis without accurate cost measurement, but including a sensitivity analysis incorporating clinically sensible variations in important variables

Level	Rx/prevention, aetiology/harm	Prognosis	Diagnosis	Economic analysis
4	Case-series (and poor quality cohort and case–control studies)	Case-series (and poor quality cohort and case–control studies)	Any of: • reference standard was not objective, unblinded or not independent; • positive and negative tests were verified using separate reference standards; • study was performed in an appropriate spectrum of patients	Analysis with no sensitivity analysis
5	Expert opinion without explicit critical appraisal, or based on physiology, bench research or 'first principles'			Expert opinion without explicit critical appraisal, or based on economic theory

Grades of recommendation:

A Level 1a to 1c
B Level 2a to 3b
C Level 4
D Level 5

[1] Systematic review with homogeneity
[2] Clinical practice guidelines

These pages have been adapted from the CEBM Levels of Evidence: http://www. cebm.net, originally created by Dave Sackett and Suzanne Fletcher and subsequently adapted by Chris Ball, Bob Philips, Brian Haynes, Sharon Straus, Martin Dawes and Paul Glasziou.
You should consult the web site for further details on how to use the levels

Study designs

This page gives a brief comparison of the advantages and disadvantages of the different types of study.
http://cebm.net

Case–control study

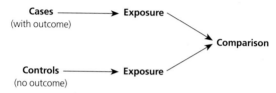

Patients who have developed a disorder are identified and their exposure to suspected causative factors is compared with that of controls who do not have the disorder. This permits estimation of odds ratios (but not of absolute risks). The advantages of case–control studies are that they are quick, cheap, and are the only way of studying very rare disorders or those with a long time lag between exposure and outcome. Disadvantages include the reliance on records to determine exposure, difficulty in selecting control groups, and difficulty in eliminating confounding variables.

Cohort study

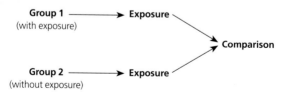

Patients with and without the exposure of interest are identified and followed over time to see if they develop the outcome of interest, allowing comparison of risk. Cohort studies are cheaper and simpler than RCTs, can be more rigorous than case–control studies in eligibility and assessment, can establish the timing and sequence of events, and are ethically safe. However, they cannot exclude unknown confounders, blinding is difficult, and identifying a matched control group may also be difficult.

Crossover design
Subjects are randomly assigned to one of two treatment groups and followed to see if they develop the outcome of interest. After a suitable period, they are switched to the other treatment. Since the subjects serve as their own controls, error variance is reduced and a smaller sample size is needed than in RCTs. However, the 'washout' period may be lengthy or unknown and crossover designs cannot be used where treatment effects are permanent.

Cross-sectional survey
Measures the prevalence of health factors (outcomes or determinants) at a point in time or over a short period. Cross-sectional studies are relatively cheap and simple to perform, as well as ethically safe. However, they cannot establish causation (only association) and are susceptible to bias (recall bias, confounding, Neyman bias).

Diagnostic validation study

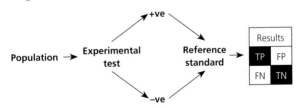

Randomized controlled trial (RCT)
Similar subjects are randomly assigned to a treatment group and followed to see if they develop the outcome of interest. RCTs are the most powerful method of eliminating (known and unknown) confounding variables and permit the most powerful statistical analysis (including subsequent meta-analysis). However, they are

expensive, sometimes ethically problematic, and may still be subject to selection and observer biases.

Index